The Better Baby Book

How to Have a Healthier, Smarter, Happier Baby

Lana Asprey, M.D.,

and

David Asprey

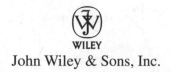

WILEY

John Wiley & Sons, Inc.

To our children, Anna and Alan,
and their children, and so on

Published by John Wiley & Sons, Inc., Hoboken, New Jersey
Published simultaneously in Canada

ISBN 978-1-118-13713-0 (paper); ISBN 978-1-118-22519-6 (ebk);
ISBN 978-1-118-23624-6 (ebk); ISBN 978-1-118-26342-6 (ebk)

Printed in the United States of America
10 9 8 7 6 5 4

This book contains references to research sources. Full references for the book may be found at www.betterbabybook.com/research.

Contents

Acknowledgments

We wrote this book because, after careful reflection, it seemed like the single best thing we could do to help the world be better. If parents learn what they can do to give their children better genes, their children will be stronger, smarter, and healthier—and then they will pass those genes on to their children. What an awesome way for a book to live on even as the printed version of these pages crumble to dust. We are grateful that we had the knowledge, education, and resources to create this program for our children. But we did not do it alone.

Gary Taubes, the author of the *New York Times* best seller *Good Calories, Bad Calories*, was kind enough to read our proposal and then introduce us to his agent, Kristine Dahl at ICM, who agreed to become our literary agent. Were it not for Gary's generosity and Kris's guidance and hard work representing us in finding a publisher, this book wouldn't have happened. Our thanks to you both, and to Laura Neely of ICM as well.

Our thanks to Andrew Clark, our researcher, who spent countless hours finding the references that we used to educate ourselves before we knew this was going to become a book. There were more than 1,300 references, to be more accurate, and Andrew formatted and posted them on our website so they will be available for everyone who has the time and desire to cull through them. His tireless attention to writing and editing was critical. This book wouldn't exist without Andrew's diligence and attention to every detail.

Ronnie Falcao, LM, MS, CPM, our homebirth midwife, shared her amazing knowledge about how birth affects baby health and wellness, and she provided gentle but insistent encouragement to write this book after she saw how transformative our program was when we used it ourselves. We are grateful that Ronnie runs gentlebirth.org, a wonderful site for parents looking to change birth into the emotional and spiritual experience it is. Barbara Findeisen, one of the world's foremost experts on pre-and perinatal psychology, also helped to shape our understanding of birth and how important it is for healthy children. Barbara can be found at starfound.org. Jan Rydfors, MD, our ob-gyn at Stanford, was amazingly open and supportive of our nontraditional approach, saying, "Whatever you're doing, keep it up. It's working!"

Our thanks to Dr. Philip Lee Miller, MD, of Los Gatos Longevity Institute (antiaging.com), who used bioidentical hormones and nutrition to help both of us balance our hormones for maximum health and fertility. Dr. Miller generously provided knowledge and support far beyond expectations, and it made a difference to us personally, and to the book and hopefully the parents who read it.

For nearly twenty years, world-class health and medical researchers and practitioners have been presenting their findings to the public at Silicon Valley Health Institute (svhi.com) meetings in Palo Alto. Dave is grateful to be president of SVHI and believes that this book would not have been possible without the knowledge he gained from more than a decade of learning with experts. In particular, Steve Fowkes, the biochemist adviser to SVHI, author of several health books, and head of CERI.com, played a pivotal role in the evolution of this book by sharing an almost supernatural understanding of the inner workings of human biochemistry.

Our editor at John Wiley & Sons, Thomas Miller, and assistant editor Jorge Amaral were hugely helpful in bringing the book to fruition and keeping our writing concise and on target. Beth Rashbaum, an independent editor, helped to set the tone of the book early in our process of writing.

The members of the Better Baby team—Andrew, Alexis, and Aaron—have all helped to pull this knowledge together, and we appreciate the passion they put into their work every day.

Dave wishes to thank Lana for so closely following this program while she was pregnant. The results of that effort play with him in our yard every day! Lana wishes to thank Dave for cooking all of those low-toxin, high-healthy-fat Better Baby meals, and most especially for making so much amazingly good, fertility-enhancing, homemade ice cream!

But most of all, we'd like to thank our parents, who did their best to pass great genes on to us. We in turn are doing our best to improve those genes and pass them down to our own children, and we sincerely hope they do the same with their children.

PART ONE

The Better Baby Plan

1

You Are a Cocreator: The Better Baby Plan

There's still much we don't understand about how the wonderful, amazingly complex little beings called babies develop and grow, even though we've been trying to figure it out from time immemorial. As part of this effort, researchers were trying to understand the role that genes play, and in the 1990s they set out to sequence the human genome. Their work led to today's understanding that our genes don't have the final word on who we are or what our children will be. Instead, our children's biological prospects are the result of a delicate interplay of environment and parental genes. This intricate dance determines which genes will be "turned on," or expressed, then passed on to the next generation, at which stage the interplay of heredity and environment again affects which genes will be turned on.

The study of the complex interaction of genes and environment is called *epigenetics*, a new field of study that, as of this writing, is only fifteen years old. New as it is, we believe it is going to forever change our basic understanding of human development and prove to be an even more exciting discovery than the decoding of the human genome.

As prospective parents who inevitably worried about the worst while hoping for the best, we had mixed feelings when we learned about early epigenetic discoveries. We were relieved, because the discoveries meant our genes would not necessarily curse our children with our shortcomings, but at the same time we were concerned that epigenetics meant we would not necessarily give our children our talents, either. The more we learned, however, the more we realized that it would be possible to tip the scales toward our "good" genes and away from our genetic weaknesses.

Countless factors can cause any of a baby's genes to turn on or off during the time in the womb. Even a mother's thoughts and feelings during pregnancy can play a significant role in determining what personality traits, characteristics, and behaviors her child may inherit. The three most common things that affect gene expression are the mother's diet and nutrition, her environment, and her emotions. Having a healthy father also has a big effect on a baby's genes, much more than many people realize.

Once we understood the implications of the new epigenetic discoveries, we decided to combine Lana's medical training with Dave's expertise in nutrition to create a program to try to turn on the healthiest genes in our children. We maximized our exposure to health-enhancing activities and substances and minimized our exposure to substances that could be harmful. We even did this before Lana got pregnant so that the womb environment would be as welcoming as possible once it was time to start our family.

So, like most health-conscious prospective parents, we exercised, got extra sleep when possible, and spent hours finding out about everything from the best crib mattress to the least toxic paint for the nursery. Beyond this, we did the in-depth medical research described earlier in order to be sure we had the best and the most current information.

Once we put our research into action, the science proved itself over and over. Lana got pregnant quickly and easily. This was a great relief, because her previous ob-gyn thought that Lana's advanced age (thirty-nine) and the fact that she had polycystic ovary syndrome made it unlikely that she would be able to get pregnant without hormone treatments or in vitro fertilization. During her pregnancy, Lana never had any morning sickness, unlike other women in her family who were so badly affected by morning sickness some had to be hospitalized.

When Lana got pregnant with our first child after six months on our program, the results of her prenatal quadruple screen blood test—which tests for four major factors in the blood that indicate neural tube defects, genetic disorders such as Down syndrome, and other chromosomal abnormalities—were better than average for her age and showed a small risk of birth defects. Naturally, we were very pleased, and the follow-up ultrasound indicated that our daughter was perfectly healthy—which proved to be the case when she was born.

With our second baby, after more than two years on the program, it was a different story.

Lana again had the early pregnancy blood tests, and this time the lab technician called our midwife to ask about what he thought was a mistake on the paperwork. He said that Lana had scored "negative times four," which is the best result possible, but that someone must have written Lana's birthday down wrong. He said, "Surely Lana is in her early twenties, not in her early forties, right? We have never seen a woman over forty with results that great." When our midwife confirmed that Lana was over forty, the lab technician's comment was "Whatever you guys are doing, keep doing it, because it's working!" Our midwife agreed (in fact, it was she who eventually convinced us to write this book). Having attended more than seven hundred births in twelve years of practice, she said that Lana was one of the healthiest pregnant women she'd ever seen, regardless of age, and that our babies were as healthy as they could possibly be.

According to Lana, who as a practicing physician has also delivered babies, both of her pregnancies were "textbook" easy. In our midwife's words, "There is very little for me to do, other than sit back and enjoy this journey with you and Dave." Our ob-gyn, who practices at Stanford Hospital in Palo Alto, California, and saw us through both pregnancies, was equally pleased and encouraging. The Better Baby Plan, which we created for our own use and now offer to you, boils down to the following four simple principles, which we call the four pillars of this book:

1. Eat the right foods.
2. Take the right supplements.
3. Detoxify your body before, during, and after pregnancy.
4. Minimize stress.

Of course, many pregnancy books tell you to eat healthy food, take a prenatal vitamin, and reduce stress. This is good advice, but there is a lot of confusion about what a healthy diet really is, which of the hundreds of prenatal vitamins on the market is best, and how to minimize stress. As you read on, you'll see that our Better Baby Plan uses the latest scientific findings to shed light on all of these issues.

The rest of this chapter will provide you with some background on the new science of epigenetics. You'll learn more about what happens at conception, how DNA actually works, and what the critical epigenetic factors are that influence your baby's development.

What Happens at Conception

Once an egg and a sperm come together, the mother's and father's genes unite to form a new cell called a *zygote*. The zygote begins *mitosis*, or cell division, and in seven days grows into a collection of cells called a *blastocyst*, which then travels down the fallopian tube and tries to attach to the wall of the uterus. If the blastocyst is successful, its cells begin to multiply and specialize. During specialization, as the cells begin to form the different parts of the baby's body, they take instructions from both their DNA and (as epigenetics has revealed) the environment.

Among the first differentiated parts to form is the neural tube, which later develops into the baby's brain and spinal cord. A newborn baby's brain contains an estimated hundred billion neurons (nerve cells), a level of complexity too high to be determined by our genetic code alone. In other words, the complexity of the brain far exceeds the capacity of its own genetic blueprint. This seems impossible, but the missing link, according to the new science of epigenetics, is the environment, which influences the genetic code and affects its interpretation.

Since primary brain structure develops in the womb, it is in the womb that environment has the most profound impact on the brain. Although DNA may dictate the basic structure for nervous-system building blocks like neurons and ganglia (nervous system tissues), the connections and relationships between neurons, which are critical to brain function, are at least in part determined by the early womb environment. So building a better brain must start in the earliest days of life.

This gives us a new perspective on the impact of toxins like cigarette smoke or alcohol during pregnancy. If these toxins damage neural networks in the early phase of a baby's brain development, they can cause birth defects to begin to form and can have lifelong effects on brain structure. As you read through this section, you'll see how even a mother's mood can have an effect on a baby's fundamental neurological makeup. The influence of the womb environment on gene translation and cell growth is responsible for many of the infinite gradations of difference that make each person unique.

It's not just your genes that make you you; it's your environment, too.

Sending Your Baby Growth-Mode Messages

To understand how the womb environment affects development, let's look carefully at DNA and its role in growth. Inside cells, genes act like an instruction manual. They contain information that teaches the cell how to build proteins, the building blocks of nearly every cell and organ in our bodies, such as muscle tissue, cell membranes, digestive enzymes, and the hormones that regulate critical body functions like sleep and wake cycles, body temperature, and weight. Proteins are also the building blocks of the signaling substances in the brain that help us to lay down memories, process information, or pull a hand away from a plate that's too hot.

Yet of all the genes in the human genome, only about 5 percent actually give instructions. The other 95 percent are *noncoding genes*; they act as on-off switches that change how the remaining 5 percent should be interpreted. Robert Sapolsky, a professor of biological sciences and urology at Stanford University, likens the human genome to a hundred-page book in which the first ninety-five pages are instructions on reading the last five pages. It is these switches that are continually turned on and off by our food, thoughts, experiences, and environment. In other words, our first ninety-five pages are rewritten on an ongoing basis!

Every time a switch is flipped, your DNA is translated just a bit differently. Sometimes these switches are changed by messenger molecules like hormones, which in turn are affected by your thoughts and emotions. Sometimes these switches are flipped by toxins or carcinogens. For example, a certain toxin may be capable of flipping a switch that results in the uncontrolled cell proliferation that turns into a cancerous tumor.

Bruce H. Lipton, a cell biologist and the author of *The Biology of Belief: Unleashing the Power of Consciousness, Matter, and Miracles*, describes a fetus as continuously "downloading" genetic information from its environment so it can develop accordingly. He notes that cells have a group reaction to the environment in which they operate together in one of two basic modes: growth or defense. When an organism is in growth mode, it absorbs nutrients, reproduces, rests, or engages in activity that enhances itself or its species. When an organism is in defense mode, however, it emphasizes processes that protect it from perceived threats, at the expense of the energy that goes into growth-mode processes.

Like every living organism, the cells that make up the child in your womb will select either growth or defense mode based on the messages they receive from the environment. Before birth, almost all of the knowledge that a baby receives about the outside world is filtered through the mother's body. This is, in effect, the baby's environment, and the baby's cells will select gene programs that the environment signals are best suited to survival. This is nature's way of preparing your baby for what he or she will face after birth.

Hormone levels have an enormous influence on the messages your baby receives and are responsible for many aspects of development. For example, having enough testosterone in the womb at a specific moment during fetal development can change your baby's life. Peter Lovatt, a psychologist at Britain's University of Hertfordshire, has found that men who were exposed to higher levels of testosterone in the womb are judged by women to be better dancers. Such men have greater control over their bodies and are more attractive as prospective partners—not just for a dance or two, but for life. In other words, the "dance floor" is tilted in their favor, and the band is playing their song!

Other desirable traits that are tied to prenatal testosterone levels—for babies of *both* sexes—are athleticism, musical ability, and facial symmetry. Studies show that facial symmetry has more of an effect than any other physical attribute on a person's appeal to prospective mates.

The body needs healthy fats to create hormones and maintain them at proper levels, which is one of the most important reasons our recommended diet is high in healthy fats.

As the prospective parent of a Better Baby, your goal is to use nutrition, environment, and stress-control techniques to send your unborn baby the message to remain in growth mode. That's what the rest of this book is about. Keeping your baby in growth mode and out of defense mode is central to a healthy pregnancy and a healthy baby, and it will affect your child's entire life. If a baby goes into defense mode, the steps that must be taken to ensure protection always come at a price. No matter how minor the defensive reaction is, it diverts energy from growth and development. Since your baby is so sensitive during critical growth phases in the womb, a defensive reaction may deprive your baby of the only chance to develop certain abilities and attributes.

The Power of Epigenetics: Our DNA Is Not Set in Stone

Scientists define epigenetics as the study of heritable changes in gene function that occur without a change in the DNA sequence. In plain English, this means that the environment affects gene translation without changing the original DNA gene sequence inside the cell. In even plainer English, it means that what we do can cause our baby's genes—and our own—to switch on or off.

There's an important type of molecule inside our cells that works with DNA called *ribonucleic acid* (RNA). DNA is an instruction manual, and RNA is responsible for reading the instructions from DNA and communicating them to other parts of the cell. These instructions control what sorts of proteins the cell will manufacture and use. Cells create protein only when RNA goes to the correct DNA strand, gets instructions from the DNA, and carries these instructions to the cell's protein-manufacturing area, known as the RER (*rough endoplasmic reticulum*).

Here's where epigenetics comes in. Think of the DNA double helix as encased in a "sleeve" of regulatory proteins, and if that sleeve allows RNA through to read the genes, those genes will be turned on. If the sleeve of regulatory proteins blocks RNA from reading the genes, those genes will be turned off. Since the environment has a large say in how the sleeve is configured, it also influences which genes RNA can get through to read.

Many different signals from the environment affect the regulatory sleeve. These signals can be chemical or electromagnetic, they can come from inside the body or outside it, and they can come from our emotions. For example, many genes in the human body are turned on or off by a person's thoughts, feelings, and experiences. These genes have a profound effect on immune function and resistance to disease. They can be activated in as little as three seconds. Holistic doctor Deepak Chopra

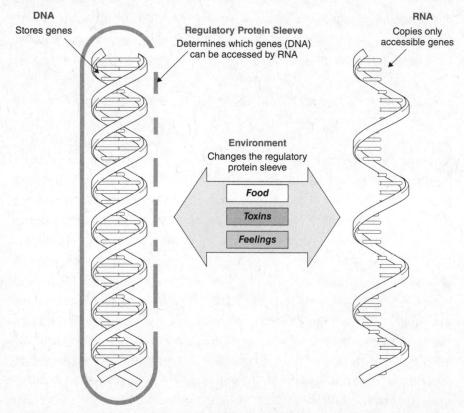

The environment controls which genes RNA can replicate (conceptual model only).

recently publicized a study showing that a short period of meditation directly affected the expression of more than five hundred genes.

Unfortunately, epigenetic effects don't always make things better. Sometimes they promote genetic programs for defense instead of genetic programs for growth. Poor habits on the part of mothers and fathers can turn on harmful genes, which are then passed on to the children. This can occur, for example, if the parents are overweight. A 2010 study at Boston's Children Hospital found that children of overweight mothers were more prone to being overweight than children of mothers with average body mass index. The older the children got, the more overweight they became.

Another example is undernourishment. If a parent is malnourished, disorders can develop that sometimes affect not just his or her children but also her children's children and beyond. Thus, a Dutch famine at the end of World War II led to higher schizophrenia rates in later generations. In the United States, researchers blame malnourishment in Southern women during the Civil War for the unusually high incidence of stroke that persisted among their descendants for several generations.

Epigenetic factors have a greater influence in the womb than at any other time in a person's life. Such factors, which include the mother's diet, environment, stress level, and emotions, can send various kinds of signals to the protein sleeve surrounding an unborn baby's DNA. Some of these signals are helpful and some are harmful, and they have a tremendous effect right after fertilization. They don't change your baby's genetic makeup, but they do (at least in part) determine which of the genes in a baby's DNA sequence will become functional. This is why we emphasize creating good health in the mother (and the father) even before conception.

To see epigenetics in action, we can look at the results of a famous Duke University study, published in *Molecular and Cellular Biology* in 2003. In this study, specially bred mice that were bright yellow and genetically susceptible to obesity, diabetes, and cancer were fed certain vitamins before and during conception and pregnancy. The resulting baby mice were healthy, natural brown-colored mice with no tendency toward obesity or disease. The vitamins and supplements given to the mother mice suppressed the bad genes that would have caused the yellow color and all the associated disease susceptibilities in their offspring.

The vitamins given to the mice included choline, trimethylglycine, folic acid, and vitamin B12—all are what are called *methyl donors*. Methyl donors can change the sleeve of proteins around the DNA in a recently fertilized egg, causing RNA to read DNA differently and have a big effect on which genes will be expressed. That's why we focus not just on food but also on prenatal supplements, and it's why we stress the importance of trying to conceive when the mother's body is optimally nourished and healthy.

Ideally, parents should also choose to conceive when the mother is not under a lot of stress. If certain stress hormones like cortisol are present in high quantities or are elevated for long periods, it can cause the body to go into the defense mode we discussed earlier. This helps cells to respond to threats more quickly, but it uses energy the body needs for other processes. Remember we said that functioning in defense mode always comes at a cost? In the long run, this faster response and higher energy use wears cells out.

In contrast, physical exercise, yoga, meditation, and prayer are all known to reset cell activity, slowing it down to its normal, more sustainable pace. Breathing exercises, relaxation training, meditation and other mindfulness techniques, good relationships with family and friends, group support, and even a healthy expression of aggression have the same reset effect. This is why they promote health and longevity. There's a good biological reason behind the advice to "take a deep breath" when you're upset—you're actually slowing your cells down and helping them to return to growth mode.

What happens in the womb isn't the only thing that has an effect on gene expression. Studies have shown that a mother's (and presumably a father's) touch and nurturing after birth can cause different genes to be turned on or off. An experiment was done with rats in which the pups of calm mothers were swapped with pups from anxious mothers, each mother raising the other's pups. The pups from anxious mothers were genetically predisposed to anxiety. The calm mothers, who licked and groomed the pups, were much better nurturers than the anxious mothers, who paid little attention to the pups. The amazing result was that the anxious pups became calm under the care of the calm mother rats. The pups' cognitive test results showed that they were more curious and that they explored new environments with less fear and hesitation. The scientists performing the experiment noted that the calm mothers' behavior caused permanent changes in the way the anxious pups' genes were translated. Based on this and other studies, there is ample evidence that a wide range of social interactions affects gene translation, especially during critical childhood development phases.

If gene translation can change after birth, imagine the power of this effect in the womb, during the most critical stages of development!

In *The Prenatal Prescription: A State-of-the-Art Program for Optimal Prenatal Care*, Peter Nathanielsz, a Cambridge University–educated doctor and expert in fetal development, gives an excellent practical example of epigenetics at work. He tells a story about two brothers.

The first brother, James, was born on a warm Southern California evening at a low-stress time in his parents' lives, when things were going well for them. Later, the father, Michael, was injured, became disabled, and lost his job as an engineer. The family moved back to its original home in Pittsburgh to be near family and old friends. The mother, Alice, kept food on the table by working at a large commercial laundry. This was a stressful environment full of noise and chemicals, and she worked there six days a week, including during her pregnancy with her second son, William, until the very day she went into labor.

James and William both grew up eating a diet typical of the Pittsburgh area: high in starch, sugar, carbohydrates, and unhealthy fats and low in proteins, healthy fats, and fresh vegetables—the same diet that causes so many health problems today. Nonetheless, James enjoyed good health, whereas William was diagnosed with high blood pressure at forty years old, contracted diabetes at fifty, and died of a stroke in his early sixties. James lived well into his eighties as a healthy man before dying of old age. The different womb environments that James and William were exposed to during critical stages of fetal development affected their whole lives.

According to Nathanielsz, how we leave the world is mostly determined by how we enter it. What happens in the womb environment can largely predict your baby's cardiovascular health, eating patterns, tendency to gain weight, emotional resilience, intelligence, susceptibility to cancer, resistance to infection, and even blood pressure. The blood pressure of women during pregnancy has been shown to correlate directly with the blood pressure of their children in adulthood.

More on Growth Mode and Defense Mode

The cells in our bodies work together in systems at least as complex as human society. Cells continuously communicate with one another, signaling other cells to either increase or decrease activity for the common good of the whole body.

If the cells of a baby in the womb face a shortage of oxygen or nutrients, they may be forced to allocate their limited resources in ways that can affect the health of that baby after birth and throughout life. This would be analogous to a farmer who harvests the corn crop and uses all of it to feed the family during a winter of severe food shortages. This helps the family to survive the winter, but afterward there is no corn to sow, and the next winter is likely to be much harder.

Similarly, if adverse conditions in the womb force a fetus to focus on short-term survival, it may have to forgo what is truly a once-in-a-lifetime opportunity for optimal development. For example, if there are inadequate supplies of nutrients or oxygen, a fetus will devote more of its resources to brain development, a shift that may come at the expense of other organs and tissues, which will no longer have an opportunity to grow properly.

The circulatory system is one of the possible victims of the shortage of resources in defense mode. If this system doesn't develop properly, there will be too few blood vessels supplying one or more of the baby's organs. A diminished blood supply means that these organs will receive less oxygen and nutrients throughout life and may not perform as efficiently as they should.

Another possible result of being in prolonged defense mode is an underdeveloped liver or digestive system. While a baby is in the womb, the mother performs all digestive and detoxifying (liver) functions for the fetus. Since these systems aren't used in utero, most fetuses give them the lowest priority if environmental factors have caused a shift into defense mode and a consequent rationing of resources. The result is that these organs may not have a chance to develop normally, eventually causing problems that cannot be reversed. No known food or supplement given to the baby after birth will be able to change the structure of an underdeveloped liver. This is why keeping your baby in growth mode and out of defense mode is so critical.

Just as babies in the womb respond to how much oxygen and nutrients cross the placenta, they are also sensitive to their mothers' stress levels, which are signaled by changes in heart rhythm, blood pressure, and sounds, as well as by certain hormones like cortisol that cross the placenta. If there are heavy loads of cortisol over a prolonged period, the message to the baby is that the outside world is a dangerous place, and the baby's whole body may enter defense mode and not develop as it should. This underdevelopment sometimes comes with lifelong effects.

Many people have heard the old saying "You are what you eat." Epigenetics shows us that you are also what you breathe, feel, and think, and these factors have a profound effect on your children, too. Epigenetics is groundbreaking because it proves once and for all that we as parents have more control over the health of our unborn children than we ever dreamed possible. The knowledge that we have this control brings with it an obligation to use that opportunity to pave the way for maximal good health in our children—starting even before conception, if possible.

2

Road Map to a Healthy Pregnancy

This chapter provides a brief overview of our program so you know what's coming and how it fits into the big picture. It is organized according to the four pillars we discussed in chapter 1 (eat right, take the right supplements, detoxify your body, and minimize stress). Although we cover many subtopics as the book progresses, you'll find it helpful to keep these four pillars in mind.

Eat the Right Foods

We make powerful dietary recommendations in chapters 4 and 5 about what to eat and what not to eat. Our recommendations, which will provide your baby with all the nutrients he or she needs to grow, are backed by the most recent epigenetic science and offer protection from toxic foods. These are the same dietary recommendations that led Lana to have no morning sickness or cravings during pregnancy, even though she was in her forties when we had our children. From a fertility stand-point, our diet enabled Lana to have two healthy babies, the second at forty-two years of age. We also share tips on how to cook food to make it healthier.

We spent time learning how to make healthy food delicious, because if food doesn't taste good, look good, smell good, and feel good, you can be sure that most pregnant women won't eat it. Many of our recipes are available online at www.betterbabybook.com.

Take the Right Supplements

We found that a shocking number of mothers—more than fifty million worldwide—have children with cognitive problems because of a lack of basic vitamins. For instance, if a mother is iodine deficient during preg-nancy, her baby's brain will not develop the best it can. Since a deficiency in iodine causes poor cognitive performance in babies, it's critical that mothers have enough iodine to avoid the problem. But "good enough" wasn't our goal—we wanted the best possible results.

Our supplements chapters will show you exactly how we not only avoided cognitive dysfunction in our children but also maximized their cognitive abilities. We spent hundreds of hours researching what works and what is safe. We found dozens of nutritional deficiencies that affect fetal development, and we realized that it was important to support our diet with nutritional supplements, including vitamins, minerals, and food isolates, as well as a few carefully selected phar-maceutical drugs.

We explain many details and fine points about supplementation, including the fact that it's sometimes key to take very specific forms of certain supplements if they're to be useful and healthy. We also found that standard supplementation with prenatal vitamins (and maybe some folic acid) is woefully inadequate, and we even discov-ered toxins in many prenatal vitamin products. You'll find everything about the supplements and drugs we used in chapters 7 and 8. If the only thing you remember from this book is that one-a-day prenatals are not enough, you'll have improved your chances of a healthy, optimal pregnancy.

Detoxify Your Body before, during, and after Pregnancy

It seems cliché to say that you need to detoxify your body. Detoxing has all the connotations of the Betty Ford Center, and the word is now so overused that average people don't seem to know what detoxing is and what it isn't. Some companies sell a pill that they claim will detox you.

Lana's experience as a physician helped her to understand how toxins affect the body, but it was Dave's expertise in nutritional approaches to health that really enabled us to focus our research on toxins, gaining an understanding of how toxins get into our bodies, where they hide, and how to remove them. There are many little-known ways that our bodies even make their *own* toxins, which cause adverse effects in fetal development. We were also able to link certain toxins with specific symptoms in babies and mothers. Much of what we reveal on this topic is unheard of in most doctors' offices.

Perhaps our most surprising topic is a class of toxins called *mycotoxins* that are produced by molds and are common in human and animal food supplies. Mycotoxins are so toxic to animal embryos that farmers actually test animal feed before giving it to pregnant animals. Many of these toxins closely resemble the primary female hormone estrogen, so they confuse the mother's and the baby's estrogen receptors, leading to early (precocious) puberty in young girls, impaired fertility in mothers, and low sperm count and shrunken testes in boys and men. Since they're hormone disrupters, these toxins have an effect at very low concentrations, even those measured in parts per billion. There are no government standards or tests required for some of these toxins, and we believe there is evidence that the current levels of them that are legally permitted in processed foods is far too high for pregnant women to be eating.

We will teach you how to spot foods that contain toxins so you can avoid them. We'll teach you how and why to keep your environment as free of toxins as possible, and we'll share the detoxification methods we developed for ourselves and our children. We'll also explain why it's important to spend time and money ensuring that you're free of low-level undiagnosed pathogenic diseases (like Lyme) before becoming pregnant.

Keeping toxins and other intruders away from your baby is vital to telling your baby that it's okay to maintain growth mode. Your own health is likely to improve dramatically, your fertility will skyrocket, and your baby will be free to grow uninhibited. See chapters 9 through 13 for all of the details.

Minimize Stress

Minimizing stress involves thinking positively and managing your emotions. The topic of emotions and stress is something many of us don't pay much attention to, but it's essential for a healthy pregnancy. That's why we'll spend extra time introducing emotions and stress right here, early in the book. As you read on, don't become dismayed that you must reduce stress and get your emotions in order right away, especially if you're already pregnant. In chapter 15 we introduce cutting-edge techniques for reducing stress. We specifically found techniques that don't take much time but produce huge results.

Science has now confirmed that what happens in the womb can have a profound, lifelong effect on a baby. In the last twenty years, Jason Birnholz, a doctor and former Harvard Medical School professor who was one of the creators of diagnostic ultrasound imaging, has taken more than fifty thousand fetal sonogram pictures. He has concluded that fetuses—especially those beyond the fourth month of pregnancy—aren't much different from newborns, in part because they display emotional reactions similar to those of babies. Science now suggests that a baby's time in the womb isn't dark and silent.

Although science has confirmed this, because we are parents it really didn't take another doctor or a Harvard professor to tell us this. Like most mothers you might ask, Lana was certain that our children were conscious while she carried them in her womb.

As a fetus develops, it experiences two levels of consciousness The first is the collective sensation of the individual molecular sensors in each cell. We usually refer to this stream of experience as subconscious. From the moment of conception, subconscious experience shapes later development and personality characteristics. Eastern beliefs and Western science combined suggest that this subconscious experience is behind some of the gut feelings and intuitive knowledge we experience as adults.

The fetus's second level of consciousness comes into being as the organized central nervous system forms, including the brain and its neurological networks. Once this happens, a fetus is constantly tuned into its mother's thoughts, feelings, and actions. The womb environment therefore shapes brain growth, personality, temperament, and even brain power from the moment of conception.

At just twenty-eight days old, when the embryo measures a quarter of an inch in diameter, the tiny blood vessel that is the precursor of the heart begins to beat, and the three primary parts of the brain have already formed. Even though consciousness isn't apparent at this time, cellular biology suggests the presence of a subconscious awareness. At six weeks, when the fetus is only half an inch long, it can respond to touch. By four months, the fetus develops curiosity about the womb environment and begins to play with the umbilical cord or suck his or her thumb. At nineteen to twenty weeks, the fetus has begun sustaining brain-wave patterns, and by twenty-two weeks, the fetus has brain patterns similar to an adult's.

During pregnancy, communication between mother and child occurs at several levels, and in both directions. Thomas Verny, a psychiatrist at the Santa Barbara Graduate Institute, describes them as sensory, molecular, and intuitive communication.

Sensory Communication

Verny reports that at five months, fetuses have been seen reacting to loud sounds by raising their arms and covering their ears, and they even react to a light flashed at the mother's abdomen. At twenty-two weeks, fetuses who tasted bitter poppy seed oil that was introduced to the womb were observed to grimace, and fetuses who tasted sweet substances swallowed amniotic fluid at twice the usual rate. During the last trimester, brain-wave studies show sustained visual and tactile sensation, and a fetus even experiences times of sleep and wakefulness. Just six months after conception, the fetus is a "sensing, feeling, aware, and remembering human being," according to Verny.

Your fetus is very sensitive. Fetuses have responded to gentle pricks to their heels with facial grimacing, clenched hands, and leg withdrawal.

Mothers and nurses caring for preterm babies frequently observe a pain response.

Given this information, what is your baby experiencing inside you? Researchers at the University of North Carolina suspended a waterproof microphone in the amniotic fluid of one mother to find out. A fetus is sensitive to sound at just nineteen weeks. At this point, your unborn baby can hear the pulse of the blood flowing through your veins, hear your stomach rumble, sense food passing through your gastrointestinal tract, and hear and remember the sound of your voice.

In a groundbreaking study, University of North Carolina psychologist Anthony DeCasper showed that newborns not only hear their mother's voices, they can also assemble sound patterns and remember what was said (not the meaning of the words, just their sound patterns). DeCasper had sixteen mothers tape their readings of three children's stories. At six and a half weeks of pregnancy, one group of women read the first story three times a day. The second group read the second story, and the third group read the third.

When the babies were born, DeCasper offered each infant a choice of the story the mother had read to him or her prenatally and another one of the stories. To find out which choice the baby made, DeCasper invented the "suckometer": a nipple on a baby bottle connected to a computer-controlled tape player. Using the suckometer, the babies could switch between two taped stories by changing their sucking speed.

Within just a few hours of birth, thirteen of the sixteen babies adjusted their sucking rhythm to hear the familiar story, Another suckometer study, conducted by Robin Panneton, a Virginia Tech psychologist, tested melodies sung by the mother to her fetus. The babies repeatedly chose the melody their mothers had sung to them over other melodies— convincing evidence of prenatal memory.

Your unborn baby can not only see, hear, taste, and feel but can remember sensations as well. When a pregnant woman caresses her abdomen, talks, or sings, she sends messages to her baby through the baby's senses. There's evidence that babies whose mothers sing lullabies to them in the womb are happier, that babies who hear classical baroque music while in the womb display natural musical ability, and that babies begin to make associations based on their mother's language and even the dialect they hear in the womb.

Sounds that unborn babies hear actually help to shape their brains, especially during periods of rapid development. Listening to classical music (especially from the baroque period) also promotes an alert, relaxed alpha brain-wave state in the mother. This boosts the mother's positive endorphins, reduces her stress-hormone levels, and promotes growth programs in her baby.

The fetus also sends messages to the mother. Whereas newborns speak to their mothers through crying, unborn babies communicate through kicking. Mothers are naturally able to tell the difference between the meanings of their baby's cries. An "I'm tired" cry is very different from an "I'm in pain" cry. In the same way, a fetus might kick lightly when he or she is happy but kick violently (and painfully for the mother!) when he or she is upset. Mothers who want their babies are far more attuned to this communication than anxious or depressed mothers who are distracted.

Molecular Communication

There's a lot going on at the molecular level. Maternal emotions and thoughts are communicated to the baby through hormones. Hormone levels change dramatically when a woman experiences different emotions, and these hormones cross the placenta and affect the fetus similarly. If the mother is stressed, more adrenaline, norepinephrine (noradrenaline), and sex hormones reach the fetus, triggering defense mechanisms in the baby at the expense of growth. If the mother is calm, adequate levels of serotonin and dopamine and lower levels of adrenaline and cortisol tell the baby that the mother is happy and at peace.

Bruce Lipton, the author of *The Biology of Belief*, described it like this: "These decisively important love/fear signals are relayed to the fetus via the blood-borne molecules produced in response to the mother's perception of her environment." He continues, "One important part of the new credo. . . is turning away from the Darwinian notion of the 'survival of the fittest' and adopting a new credo, the survival of the most loving."

Intuitive Communication

Beyond sensory and molecular communication, there is a special connection between mother and baby during pregnancy that has been described by countless mothers, who believe they "just know" what is happening with their babies. This doesn't go only for mothers, either; fathers communicate with their unborn children at the sensory level and the intuitive level. They can also interact at the molecular level by supporting the mother emotionally and doing all they can to keep her stress levels low.

One of the keys to a successful pregnancy is realizing that your baby is sensing and feeling from the very moment of conception and that these sensations and feelings change how your baby grows. We said *conception*, not *birth*. How your baby perceives the womb environment plays an integral role in his or her development. Although your fetus may not have full sensory capacities like hearing or seeing until a few months after conception, what you say, think, breathe, eat, and feel has a huge effect even before the senses develop.

Psychologists who study intelligence know that there is a complex interaction between intelligence and emotional development. For us, doing the best we could for our children meant not only having a smarter baby but also having an emotionally healthy baby, who can grow up to become an emotionally healthy adult. There was a time in both of our lives when we'd have read that sentence and thought, "What? Babies can't even remember what happens to them at birth—this is ludicrous." We would have been wrong.

We were fortunate to learn that this was wrong before we had children. The person we thank most for showing us the facts is Barbara Findeisen, the president of the Association for Pre- and Perinatal Psychology and Health. In the last fifty years, psychological research has uncovered overwhelming evidence of this view. Findeisen herself has spent more than thirty years in the field, and through the Star Foundation, she's helped thousands of people to understand how their own births affected their physical and mental well-being. It is a repeatable phenomenon measurable by science.

A New Way of Thinking

The line of thinking we've described sounds a bit New Age, but we're certain it made a difference in the emotional health of our children, and we know that emotional health leads to better gene expression. The hardest part of keeping your unborn baby in growth mode is managing your emotions to minimize stress. A loving and peaceful womb environment triggers growth programs in a baby. Try as she may, an anxious or a depressed mother who faces an uncomfortable situation at home or financial uncertainty in her life will have a difficult time keeping her feelings away from her baby.

In our book, we describe the best methods we know for reducing stress, including breathing techniques, exercise, heart rate variability training, meditation, and yoga. Practicing a stress-reducing technique you're comfortable with will help to fill you with peace and love before and during pregnancy. We let you know the science behind each technique.

Comparing Your Baby to Others

If all of what we've written so far seems overwhelming, or if you're already pregnant and wondering how much it matters that you didn't detox before you got pregnant, we have a word of advice for you: relax. Every day, thousands of babies are born healthy in spite of their mothers eating suboptimal diets, being exposed to toxins, or being stressed out.

In this book we present every technique we found and used to make the best pregnancy possible. We didn't use some of the techniques when we had our first child, Anna. We did further research and used some of them only with our second child, Alan. Choose the techniques that feel right for you and your baby, and implement them as you see fit. And remember, even if you don't do them perfectly or you "cheat" occasionally, the odds are high that your baby will be happy and healthy if you follow the core principles.

Remember too that there is no way to compare your baby to other babies. No one can determine which parents did a better job of optimizing, because the interplay of genetics, environmental factors, and uncontrollable circumstances is too complex to analyze now. Even if you do not compare your baby to others, there is no way to be sure that your pregnancy optimization planning had any effect at all. Maybe it's just good genetics, blind luck, providence, karma, or fate. It's your call.

Even though we couldn't measure our results precisely, we decided to do our best without taking unnecessary risks, and we couldn't be happier with the results. We're convinced that our program was helpful to our entire family in tangible ways. There's no way to prove that our children are any different now than they would have been if Lana had eaten toxic processed food every day of her pregnancy. Even though we can't prove it, though, we know—the way only a mommy and a daddy can know—that our children are better off because of our efforts. We sincerely hope our book helps you to improve your baby's health, intelligence, and well-being.

Before We Continue

In the next chapter we start to describe the Better Baby Plan in detail. Before we do that, we'd like to acknowledge that there's a lot of conflicting information out there. Sometimes scientific studies aren't carried out in the most honest or effective way or are funded by special interests. Statistics are sometimes skewed and misrepresented. One study's conclusions conflict with another study's conclusions, and researchers highlight the flaws in the methodology used by other researchers. Some of the most helpful new groundbreaking research gets suppressed because it disagrees with a whole generation of scientists who didn't use newer tools when they formed their conclusions years ago.

Sometimes we present information and sources that conflict with conventional health advice. We cite many scientific studies, as well as books, articles, and websites that helped us to reach our conclusions about how to have the healthiest children we could.

We don't consider our recommendations to be comprehensive, and we don't think you should, either. New things are discovered every day. What we do know is that the information we gleaned from our sources added up to a brilliantly successful program for us. Although some might argue with the information we present, we think the success of our program is a powerful testimony to the credibility of our recommendations. We tell you exactly what we did and explain our reasons for doing it. Our program worked wonderfully for us, and we think it can work wonderfully for you, too.

When we created our plan, our goal was to take our knowledge of epigenetics and its implications for pregnancy and fetal development and use it to do the best we could. We did it for our children—and for their children and beyond. Knowing about epigenetics before we had kids taught us that many generations can be affected by what we think and do. There's good evidence that healthier, more intelligent people enjoy greater success throughout life, and we know from epigenetics that a good start lasts more than a lifetime.

PART TWO

The
Better Baby
Diet

3

Better Baby
Building Blocks

Most parents know intuitively that the most important building block for a baby is a parent's unconditional love. As scientists, we believe that the most important thing you can do as a parent is to consciously show your baby—from the moment you learn you're pregnant—that he or she is wanted and loved. Parents are biologically wired to feel this way already, and since you're reading this book, the odds are high that your baby is already benefiting from your love and desire to do everything you can for him or her.

You'll find more about the connection between emotions and Better Babies later on. For now, let's look at the physical building blocks of a baby's body and brain, which are a mix of water, healthy fats, proteins, minerals, and a few carbohydrates.

What Bodies Are Made Of

It's possible for our bodies to convert an amazing variety of foods into these basic building blocks. However, the fields of biochemistry, medical science, and nutrition show that it's much easier for our bodies to convert some foods into building blocks than others. If we provide ourselves with foods that take a lot of metabolic energy to transform them into healthy building blocks, we end up wasting that energy instead of using it to make a healthier baby.

In our quest to provide our babies with the best possible conditions for growth, we consciously chose to eat the foods that were easiest for a mother's body to convert into building blocks. This principle, along with years of medical training and research into nutrition, shapes the Better Baby nutrition plan.

In this section, we describe the basic building blocks of the human body. Although the precise ratios of the types of building blocks vary based on sex, race, age, and even individual makeup, the building blocks themselves are the same. In the next section, we'll cover the building

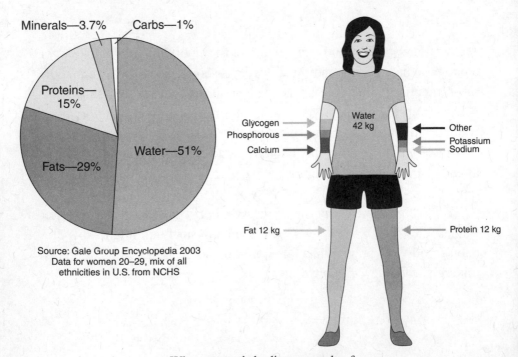

Source: Gale Group Encyclopedia 2003
Data for women 20–29, mix of all
ethnicities in U.S. from NCHS

What women's bodies are made of

blocks of the brain in particular, because building a healthy brain is one of the most important tasks.

Water

Believe it or not, water is the most common building block. The adult body is typically between 50 and 60 percent water, but newborns are 78 percent water. Most of the time, we don't pay much attention to water. But when we don't get enough and we become dehydrated, our bodies don't work well at all, especially our reproductive organs. The body can live much longer without food than it can without water, but your goal as a parent is to make sure you don't run low on either one.

Staying hydrated with purified water is essential during pregnancy, especially during the formation of amniotic fluid. Properly hydrated tissues help a mother's body to flush away toxins, so water is not only a building block for your baby, it's a way of protecting him or her from toxins. Pure water is also vital to fertility because it keeps the womb hydrated and the menstrual cycle running smoothly.

At twenty-eight weeks, a fetus is made of 84 percent water. Babies don't have fruit juice, sports drinks, or soda circulating in their bodies. These drinks aren't building blocks! Our goal is to provide the body with the things that are easiest to convert into healthy babies, and with clean water, no conversion at all is necessary. In the case of those other drinks, the body has to do a lot of work to get pure water out of them, and sometimes they even promote dehydration.

Mild chronic dehydration is surprisingly common, because people make the mistake of choosing sweetened drinks over water. In our experience, most women who switch to water and herbal teas don't have difficulty with mild dehydration anymore, and they naturally drink the amount they need. Guidelines based on number of glasses of water per day are woefully inadequate, because the body's need for water varies, especially during pregnancy.

Frequently, tap water and even many bottled waters contain harmful contaminants. Even though contaminated water meets the body's basic need for water, well-filtered water or clean mineral water meets the need with no downside. If 84 percent of your baby is water, and 51 percent of the mother is water, you want it to be clean water. We'll tell you exactly how to get clean water in chapter 10.

Fats

Women naturally carry more fat than men—about 50 percent more as a percentage of body weight. Women carry this fat (about 29 percent of body weight) because it's necessary for fertility, temperature regulation, and shock absorption. Fat is also a building block of healthy cell walls and hormones. Some fats are also healthy fuel for the body.

Fats have gained a bad reputation from the media, but many fats are healthy and essential for life. There certainly are unhealthy fats that can cause health problems. But many mothers make the mistake of "throwing the baby out with the bathwater" when they assume that eating less fat will make them or their babies healthier.

In fact, if you take away the water, a woman's body is made up of about 60 percent fat—more than twice as much fat as protein. Healthy fats are a major component of the human body, and it's very important for a pregnant woman to eat them daily. Her baby needs them badly—especially for brain growth. In fact, between twenty-eight weeks and birth, a female fetus increases the amount of fat in her body by twelve and a half times, a far bigger increase than for protein. Much of this increase comes from the fats that make up the brain itself, and the quality of the initial fat building blocks can affect brain function forever.

Our livers use healthy fats to make cholesterol when we need it. Our bodies then use the cholesterol as a building block for cell walls and hormones and even to bind to and excrete some toxins that are harmful to a growing baby. Cholesterol is a fundamental brain component—we can't live without it.

Omega fats, especially omega-3, are nutritionally essential because the body needs them to function yet cannot make them. They have to be in our diet in the proper ratios and amounts. Some of these omega fats are used in the brain to support and protect the neurons, but others in excess can lead to inflammation and health problems. Babies need the right amounts of omega fats to support brain growth.

Since our bodies are made of fats, a low-fat diet is almost always a bad idea, especially during pregnancy, when your body is trying to build another little body. We assure you that eating the right fats—the kinds bodies are made of—doesn't promote weight gain at all and won't pose a health risk. Since eating healthy fats helps the body to build the right hormones, weight *loss* is a common result. Better hormone function is also why healthy fats increase fertility.

Saturated fats are some of the best building-block fats. A whopping 90 percent of the fats in a newborn baby are saturated or monounsaturated. Healthy saturated fats are critical for a baby's brain growth. In fact, the placenta often chooses to allow saturated fats to reach the baby while blocking other fats. In chapter 4, we explain which fats your baby needs most and which foods contain them.

Proteins

Proteins are the primary structural building blocks of our bodies. They come in all shapes and sizes. The body uses proteins to make most body tissues, including bones, tendons, cartilage, muscles, internal organs, skin, and hair. The average adult is 20 percent protein, but the average woman is 15 percent protein. Like fats, proteins are not all created equal. Some proteins are easy to digest, whereas others are difficult for the body to handle. An example of easily digested protein is beef or lamb from healthy animals. Difficult proteins include gluten from wheat, casein from cow's milk, and soy.

It makes sense that meat from animals is the natural protein source closest to our own makeup. Our bodies can use other protein types, but it takes a lot more enzymes and biological energy to digest them. With meat, most of the work has already been done for us, and meat usually comes with easily used fat that is similar to our own. This is why we recommend eating meat from healthy animals during pregnancy.

Eating red meat probably goes against the health advice you've read. This advice is based on meat from animals that were raised incorrectly and fed the wrong feed. Studies of the health benefits of meat from cattle and lambs that ate the right feed (that is, grass) show that healthy red meat is one of the best choices for a pregnant woman. We'll explain this fully in chapter 5.

Between twenty-eight weeks and birth, a male fetus increases the amount of protein in his body by five times. Your baby will need the right amount—and type—of protein to grow into the healthiest baby he or she can be. A diet deficient in easily digestible protein may result in lower birth weight, lower cognitive function in the baby, or other complications.

It's our experience that most pregnant women don't eat enough protein, and much of the protein they do eat has been made very difficult for the body to use because it's gone through a chemical process called *denaturation*. Denaturation is what happens when proteins are exposed to high heat or pressure that permanently alters their structure. Denatured protein is at best hard for the body to use, and at worst it can be harmful to mother and baby. We identify which foods contain healthy protein and which foods contain harmful protein in chapters 4 and 5. We also explain how the way you cook protein makes a huge difference in how healthy it is.

Minerals

A fertile woman's body is about 4 percent minerals, with skeletal calcium, phosphorus, and potassium composing most of it, followed by magnesium, chlorine, iodine, iron, sodium, and sulfur. The body also contains trace amounts of chromium, cobalt, copper, manganese, molybdenum, selenium, vanadium, zinc, and others. These minerals perform many functions in the body and are building blocks of important enzymes and hormones.

They're required for life, and they must be kept in careful balance. Iodine composes a minuscule percentage of the body, but without it, thyroid function declines, and brain function follows. Another example of maintaining balance is the ratio of calcium to magnesium. We've all been led to believe that calcium stops osteoporosis, but the truth is that calcium by itself, without magnesium, can cause problems, including osteoporosis. Few people know that prenatal vitamins are woefully inadequate in establishing and maintaining the mineral levels that mother and baby really need. We show you how to get the minerals you need in chapter 7.

Salt

Even though only 0.15 percent of the body is salt (sodium chloride), we cannot live without it. Our bodies have incredibly sensitive mechanisms in place to regulate our salt levels, because the ratio of sodium to potassium has to be perfect at all times or, simply put, life isn't possible.

Our bodies can go to great lengths to keep sodium and potassium balanced, but there's a lot we can do to make the job easier.

It's commonly believed that eating salt leads to high blood pressure, but the science shows that only a small percentage of people with high blood pressure react strongly to salt. Michael Alderman, a past president of the American Society of Hypertension, conducted a well-controlled, four-year study of three thousand people and found that study participants who ate the least salt had the most heart attacks and cardiac complications. He concluded, "The more salt you eat, the less likely you are to die," because low-salt study subjects were less healthy and died more often than high-salt subjects. Low-sodium diets raise LDL (bad) cholesterol, reduce sex drive, and raise insulin resistance (a precursor to diabetes), all of which tilt the balance away from having the healthiest baby you can.

For healthy people, salt alone does not cause high blood pressure. High blood pressure is just as easily caused by too little calcium, magnesium, or potassium as by excess sodium. This is why reducing salt intake hasn't helped with high blood pressure, as people thought it would. It's much easier—and healthier—to deal with hypertension by increasing magnesium and potassium intake instead of reducing salt intake.

Also, sodium and salt are not the same thing. What we usually call table salt is now a mix of chemically extracted pure sodium and toxic aluminum anticaking agents. Too much sodium makes you thirsty because your body needs water to deal with the excess. Other common symptoms of excess pure sodium are cellulite, rheumatism, arthritis, gout, kidney stones, and gallstones.

High-quality sea salts, on the other hand, naturally contain a blend of minerals that provide the sodium the body needs while maintaining mineral balance. Some table salts are iodized, but iodizing doesn't even come close to getting the mineral balance right. The best salt we've found is pink salt mined in Utah or the Himalayas. These salts come from ancient seabeds that do not contain modern pollutants, but any sea salt contains a healthier mix of minerals than table salt. Prepared foods usually contain refined salt that is pure sodium, but as long as you maintain adequate magnesium and potassium intake, blood pressure is unlikely to be a problem for you, although the chemicals added to refined salt are toxic in themselves.

Energy Tip

Drinking half a teaspoon of sea salt mixed in a large glass of water right after you wake up is a great way to raise your energy level in the morning. When we wake up, our bodies are struggling to push our potassium levels down and our sodium levels up. Our adrenal glands are involved in this process. Eating a balanced salt makes the job easier for the adrenals and frees them up to increase energy levels and prepare for the day. Doing this helped Lana feel much better during pregnancy.

Our bodies naturally contain salt, and sea salts are healthy and maintain the mineral balance our bodies need. You can tell if a salt is balanced or not by seeing if you get thirsty after eating it. You may notice that you get thirsty from ordinary table salt— we certainly do. We also noticed that we can eat plenty of Himalayan salt and *not* get thirsty. This is because the minerals are more balanced.

Carbohydrates

About 1 percent of the human body is carbohydrates. This means that carbs, by themselves, are not the best building block for your baby, because your baby is not made of them. It's possible for your body to convert carbs into fats and proteins, but the energy required for that conversion would be better used directly for your baby's growth. Carbs include sugars, starches, and fiber. Grains, potatoes, breads, pastas, and sweets are mostly carbohydrates.

We'll discuss choosing (and avoiding many) carbs in chapters 4 and 5, but the bottom line is that carbs satisfy us for a very short time because they aren't what our bodies want in a food. They make us full for a short time, but we'll quickly want to eat more—especially more carbs. This starts a repetitive cycle of carbohydrate intake and stops us from eating the good fats and proteins our bodies and our babies really need. It also exposes a baby to big fluctuations in insulin, potentially setting him or her up for diabetes later in life.

Today the United States has epidemics of diabetes and obesity. Some of this is linked to an excessive intake of refined carbs in the U.S. food supply. For your baby's sake, pregnancy is one of the most important times not to be diabetic or obese.

What Brains Are Made Of

The diagram below shows what brains are made of. Like the rest of the body, the brain is mostly made of water. Skeletal muscle is about 75 percent water, for example, whereas the brain is 77 percent. The next largest component of the brain is fat (12 percent, with lots of cholesterol), followed by protein (8 percent), and a minimal amount of minerals and carbohydrates.

Healthy fats are critical to a healthy brain, and making a new brain for your baby is next to impossible without them. Cholesterol is used heavily throughout the brain. The brain also needs a lot of choline, a nutrient that is attached to healthy fats. Growing brains also need plenty of essential omega fats. To supply a baby's growing brain, the concentrations of certain omega-3 and omega-6 fats are three to four

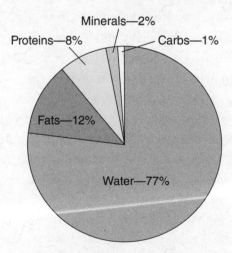

What brains are made of

times higher in a healthy newborn than they are in adults. These omega-3 and omega-6 fats are used in cell membranes and in special signaling molecules in the brain and the nervous system, but they still make up a small percentage of the total fat in the brain.

Fetuses don't store much fat until the third trimester, when they begin storing fat rapidly, most of it saturated and monounsaturated. Unlike adults, babies aren't storing the types of fat burned for energy—they're storing the types that will continue to build their brains. Your baby is storing this healthy fat to make sure that brain building blocks are available for him or her after birth. This shows how essential it is to eat plenty of healthy fats throughout pregnancy and while nursing.

The protein in the brain includes some very special amino acids. Amino acids are the building blocks of protein. Some important brain amino acids are glutamine, gamma-aminobutyric acid (GABA), and carnitine. Glutamine helps muscles grow and fuels the brain. Supplementing with it does wonders for tired mothers and fathers. GABA is both an amino acid and a neurotransmitter (a substance that transmits nerve impulses). Carnitine is an amino acid that fuels brain function and the growth of new neurons. We explain how to work glutamine, carnitine, and other supplements into your diet in chapter 7.

The brain is only 1 percent carbohydrates. Much of this is glycogen, which brain cells quickly burn for energy. Glycogen is central to proper brain function, but a low-carb diet provides enough glycogen for optimal brain function because our bodies can convert protein into glycogen. Although the brain needs some carbs, it doesn't need a lot, and it doesn't benefit from high-carb diets.

For a baby's growing brain to get the support it needs, there are two key brain components that the diet has to support: ganglia and neurotransmitters. Dendrites connect individual neurons (brain cells), which allow us to learn and become better problem solvers. Neurotransmitters are chemicals that brain cells use to communicate with one another. Some neurotransmitters you might have heard of are GABA, serotonin, and dopamine. Once the dendrites connect two neurons, the neurons can use the neurotransmitters to talk to one another. Anything that encourages new neurons to form or ganglia to grow and connect them is likely to be great for a baby's growing brain. Chapters 5 and 7 explain exactly what foods and supplements you need to support ganglia and neurotransmitters.

We have explained brain makeup to show that the brain is made of the exact same things as the rest of the body—it's almost all water, fats, and proteins. The same diet that supports a baby's growing body supports the baby's brain, too. And with all the developments in neuroscience in the past fifty years, we can even give the brain an extra boost by adding special fats and amino acids the brain needs to work its best.

If you're on statin medications to lower your cholesterol, it's important you get off the drugs before pregnancy. Low cholesterol in mothers can serve to prevent fetal brain growth. Babies are made of cholesterol that comes from mothers!

What Bodies Are Not Made Of

For the healthiest, most intelligent baby possible, the most important thing to remember is that our food should contain the same things that we're made of: mostly water, healthy fats, proteins, and minerals, along with some vegetables containing vitamins and fiber. A lot of the foods in your local grocery store aren't made of these things at all, though. The foods in your local store often contain harmful fats, denatured proteins, and too many carbohydrates. On top of that, harmful chemical additives, artificial colorings, preservatives, pesticides, fungicides, and heavy metals like mercury are common. None of those belong in a baby's body, and all of them have a negative impact on a baby's development.

When something goes into our bodies, we break it down and use it or excrete it. Much of the time, things that aren't supposed to be there don't just do nothing, they cause harm as we break them down. As parents, we wanted to make sure that the right things were there for our babies and that the wrong things weren't. The next chapter advises you on what not to eat, and that's followed by a chapter that advises you on what is good for you to eat

The old adage "You are what you eat" is precisely true, physically speaking—the foods we eat turn into our bodies. The point of this chapter has been that it takes nothing more than common sense to build a healthy baby. We humans know instinctively that we should eat foods that our bodies can use. We have presented the facts in this chapter to show why a good diet is so important: we eat things that are easy for our bodies to use and avoid foods our bodies aren't made of.

Some medical doctors, health-care professionals, and nutritionists disapprove of the diet we advocate, despite the large volume of supporting research. Yet this diet makes perfect sense to us not only because of the research but also because it has made us, our babies, and our friends who have tried it noticeably healthier and happier than any alternative diet we or they have tried. When you cast aside oversimplified headlines, the preponderance of evidence in human nutrition supports our principles.

In the coming chapters, we will describe a precise plan for providing your body with everything it needs to run properly and make a baby at the same time—at least everything we know of. Greater advances will surely be made in the future. But for now, the latest research and science is described right here in this book.

4

What Not to Eat

Here is the Better Baby approach to cooking:

- Cook slowly on low heat.
- Avoid blackening and charring.
- Cook with oils made of saturated fats and avoid cooking with monounsaturated or polyunsaturated fats.
- Avoid pasteurization, especially pasteurized dairy products.
- Eat a large percentage of your diet raw. It's healthy, and it protects your body from the harmful aspects of cooked foods.

Now let's take a look at what foods not to eat.

Fried or Overcooked Food

There are several reasons to avoid fried and overcooked foods:

- Most fats oxidize when heated. (Why this is bad is explained in the following section.)

- Proteins denature (become malformed) when heated.
- Cooking often produces harmful mutagens (agents that produce mutations).
- Cooking can cause a Maillard reaction (also explained in the following sections).
- Cooked food is harder to digest.

Oxidation

Frying and grilling usually oxidizes food—at least some parts of it. This includes panfrying, grilling, and especially deep frying. When food oxidizes, it's actually mixing chemically with the oxygen in the air. The result is that the oxygen in the air steals (oxidates) negatively charged electrons from the food molecules. When this happens, the molecules that lost electrons become ionic and frantically search for replacement electrons. These frantic searchers are called *free radicals*.

The result is that fried or overcooked food is positively charged. Since the molecules in the food are striving to balance their charges, when that food is eaten, it will steal electrons from the molecules of the body. When the molecules that make up the body lose electrons to the overcooked food, they also become imbalanced and positively charged, and a chain reaction ensues. Entire cells can die from this, and even a mass killing of cells can result. If this process is not stopped, the chain reaction can be the beginning of inflammation, cancer, and degenerative disease.

Many health foods mitigate free radical activity because they contain antioxidant molecules. Antioxidants donate electrons to free radicals without becoming free radicals themselves. Vitamin C, vitamin E, and omega-3 fatty acids are powerful antioxidants. Free radicals are satiated when their stolen electrons are returned to them, and they stop searching. The result is called *reduction*, the addition of electrons to a molecule, which is the opposite of *oxidation*, when electrons are stolen.

There are visible signs of oxidation that can help you to avoid oxidized foods. An example of very gentle oxidation is the brown color that appears on the interior of fruit (such as an apple) when it is exposed to the air. Many things oxidize just from air exposure; they don't even need heat. The charring or blackening that happens to food as it fries or grills indicates more severe oxidation. Any discoloration in the direction of brown or black is a telltale sign.

Denatured Protein

Proteins become denatured (malformed) when heated. When proteins are denatured, they're often less useful and can even be harmful to the body. The milk protein casein is a good example: once heated, casein becomes inflammatory inside the body. Any type of cooking can cause protein to denature—all it takes is heat. Denatured protein is one reason we recommend cooking lightly and at a low temperature, avoiding pasteurized products, and using only cold-processed protein supplements.

Mutagens

Cooking food produces mutagens. Mutagens are molecules that alter DNA in living cells and increase the risk of the cell becoming cancerous. Mutagens have been found even after gentle broiling and appear to be unavoidable. Raw vegetables have been shown to counteract mutagenic activity, and they also have antioxidant properties. The main idea here is to eat plenty of raw food with your lightly cooked food.

Maillard Reaction

During cooking, a chemical process known as the Maillard reaction can occur between carbohydrates and proteins. These reactions produce Maillard reaction products (MRPs), which include inflammatory carcinogens called *heterocyclic amines*. Cooking foods like milk that contain plenty of carbs and proteins together can easily result in MRPs. Gentle cooking produces fewer MRPs than faster cooking at higher heat (overcooking).

Difficult Digestion

Overcooked food strains the digestive system, which then needs more metabolic energy to operate. The brain and the digestive system end up competing for metabolic energy. Food that's harder to digest decreases the amount of energy the body could otherwise devote to brain function, development, learning, and memory. Eating raw and lightly cooked food leaves more energy for your baby to develop.

Genetically Modified Foods

When a food is genetically engineered, the source plant or animal's genes have been directly altered, making it a genetically modified organism (GMO). GMO foods are now very common. Typical GMO crops include canola, corn, cottonseed, and soybeans. In some cases, most of the supply is now GMOs, including 91 percent of soybeans and 60 percent of corn. Products that are made from these GMO crops include canola, corn, cottonseed, and soy oils; maltodextrin; most soy lecithins; and high-fructose corn syrup. Some zucchini, yellow squash, papaya, rennet (used to make cheese), and aspartame are also GMOs. GMO sugar beets are in use in the United States.

The research evidence against GMO food consumption is overwhelming. Jeffrey Smith, author of *Genetic Roulette: The Dangers of GMOs*, wrote that GMO foods have been "linked to toxic and allergic reactions, sick, sterile, and dead livestock, and damage to virtually every organ studied in lab animals." In humans, GMO foods have been linked to autoimmune disorders, inflammation, and severe food allergies. Research has led entire countries like France, Germany, and New Zealand to ban GMO farming and foods.

GMO foods have become common only in the last twenty years. It's no coincidence that during that time, the U.S. population has suffered a 400 percent increase in allergies, a 300 percent increase in asthma, a 400 percent increase in attention-deficit/hyperactivity disorder (ADHD), and a 1,500 percent increase in other autism spectrum disorders. Food-related illness doubled between 1994 and 2001. Soy began to be genetically modified in 1996. In 1996 alone, soy allergies increased by 50 percent, and soy became one of the top ten allergens in the nation.

In the United States, GMO products are not required to be labeled as such. One way to avoid them is to avoid products that contain typically GMO crops and derivative substances, which have been listed above.

Unfortunately, the number of GMO foods in the United States seems to be growing every day. Even as we were writing this book, a plan for GMO salmon was announced. It's necessary to check almost every food you buy.

The only fail-safe way to avoid GMO products is to eat certified U.S. Department of Agriculture (USDA) organic foods. At the time we wrote this book, for a food to be certified USDA organic, it had to be GMO-free. But we can't guarantee that this will always be true.

An easy way to check produce is to glance at the price lookup sticker. If the sticker contains a four-digit number, the product was conventionally grown. This usually means that synthetic fertilizers and pesticides were used, but it doesn't necessarily mean that the product is a GMO. If the sticker contains a five-digit number beginning with an 8, the product is a GMO, and you should avoid it. If the sticker contains a five-digit number beginning with a 9, it's an organic product and has never been exposed to synthetic fertilizers, pesticides, growth hormones, irradiation, or antibiotics, and it contains no GMO ingredients. That's what you want.

Unhealthy Fats

Throughout this book we recommend eating a diet high in healthy fats. This section is about the fats you'll definitely want to avoid. It helps to understand the differences between different types of fats. *Saturated* simply means that a fat is very stable in air and heat and won't turn rancid very easily. Butter, coconut oil, and animal fat from healthy animals are largely saturated. *Unsaturated fats* easily become rancid when exposed to oxygen or heat. *Polyunsaturated fats* like canola and corn oil (known as omega-6 oils) are extremely unstable and should be minimized. Monounsaturated fats like olive oil are great to eat but break down easily when cooked. *Hydrogenation* is the industrial process of chemically turning any oil into one that is heat stable but damaged. Hydrogenation is the process that makes trans-fats.

All of this matters because you should avoid eating oxidized oils before and during your pregnancy.

Cooking Oils

Most cooking oils, including canola, corn, cottonseed, peanut, safflower, soybean, sunflower, and vegetable (hereafter called "bad oils"), are unhealthy, especially when they're heated for cooking. There are four reasons to avoid bad oils and any product that contains them:

1. Many of these oils are made from crops that are commonly contaminated with mycotoxins (toxins produced by molds). Any oil containing corn or peanuts is at the highest risk for contamination.

2. Many of the oils are GMOs; that is, they are made from genetically modified crops, with canola, corn, and soy being the most likely.

3. The types of fats in these oils promote inflammation and disease inside the body. They also oxidize easily and so do even more damage when they've been used for cooking.

4. Many of the fats are synthetically hydrogenated, especially when they're included in packaged baked goods like crackers and cookies.

Bad oils contain two kinds of bad fat. The first is excessive levels of omega-6 polyunsaturated fat, which is found in all of them. The second is trans fat, which is contained in any hydrogenated oil. When you find these oils bottled in the supermarket for sale, they won't usually be hydrogenated. But many of these oils are hydrogenated before they're used in packaged food products like crackers and cookies.

Omega-6 fatty acids aren't harmful in themselves. In fact, the body needs some of them. Things go wrong with omega-6 for two reasons. First, omega-6 oxidizes very easily. Exposure to sunlight is all it takes sometimes. Second, omega-6 promotes imflammation and disease when we eat too much of it without eating enough omega-3. Experts have estimated that during most of human history, the ratio of omega-6 to omega-3 fats in the human diet was about one to one. The ratio in the modern American diet ranges between twenty to one and fifty to one! Excess omega-6 intake has been linked to cancer in numerous studies. Our diet provides all of the unoxidized omega-6 and omega-9 fats you need while being very rich in unoxidized omega-3. Omega-6 and omega-9 are so common in foods that we recommend avoiding any "healthy" omega-6 supplements like evening primrose oil.

Checklist for Avoiding Bad Oils

- Don't cook with them at home. Instead, use oils made of saturated fats, which don't oxidize as easily as monounsaturated and polyunsaturated fats. Good cooking fats are butter, coconut oil, palm oil, lard or bacon fat from pastured pigs, and tallow from grass-fed cows. We don't include chicken fat here for reasons we'll explain in chapter 5, and even though olive oil is a healthy oil, we don't recommend cooking with it (also explained in chapter 5).

- Avoid products in the grocery store that list these oils as ingredients, especially if they're hydrogenated or partially hydrogenated. You'll find them in everything from baked goods to canned protein shakes to margarine. Almost all margarines are made of bad oils; margarine is *not* healthier than butter—in fact, it's far worse.

- Avoid restaurant food that contains bad oils. This is very difficult—unhealthy oils are extremely common in restaurants, and the waitstaff often won't know the exact ingredients. During pregnancy, we pretty much avoided restaurants or asked for lightly grilled fish or steamed vegetables tossed in butter or real olive oil.

Synthetically Hydrogenated Trans Fat

When oils are used in baked goods like candies, cookies, crackers, and other snack products, manufacturers often synthetically hydrogenate or partially hydrogenate them. This is done so that the fats are stable in packaging and don't turn to liquid and leak in warm temperatures. Unfortunately, synthetic trans fats have been identified as the cause of countless health problems, including cancer. The most infamous and unhealthy trans fat of all is partially hydrogenated soybean oil.

Trans fat is dangerous because the body mistakes it for real fat and uses it to construct and maintain cell walls. The trouble is, trans fat is more rigid than natural fat. Cell walls made of trans fat are no longer flexible and porous enough for the cell to function properly. A host of new malformed cells are born, and the previously exiting cells are injured. If a pregnant or nursing mother eats trans fat, it will be used to make her baby, which presents all of the same dangers.

The research evidence against trans fat is so indisputable that if a product contains trans fat, the manufacturer is required to notify consumers on the product packaging. Beware of advertising that claims the product contains no trans fat—the Food and Drug Administration (FDA) allows packaging to claim that a product contains no trans fat even when the trans-fat content is up to half a gram per serving. Armed with this information, you can be sure that if any hydrogenated oil is in the ingredients list, the product definitely contains trans fat. Any amount of trans fat is too much—it's just too damaging to health.

Nevertheless, even though synthetic man-made trans fats aren't healthy, some natural trans fats are. Conjugated linoleic acid is a healthy natural trans fat found in butter from grass-fed cattle.

Sugar and Excess Carbohydrates

Avoiding excess sugar and carbohydrate intake is important during pregnancy and any time of life. Not only is sugar a short-lived source of energy that results in fatigue, sugar disrupts brain and hormone function and promotes obesity, infertility, and birth defects.

Sugar Is a Poor Energy Source

Eating sugar creates a cycle of highs and lows in the blood sugar and insulin levels. Insulin is a hormone secreted by the pancreas to regulate blood sugar. When you eat sugar, your blood sugar level rises, and your pancreas responds by secreting insulin. The pancreas usually overestimates how much insulin to release, especially when you eat lots of sugar at once. The insulin surge causes a fast drop in blood sugar, which renews the craving for sugar. This is one way that sugar is addictive. We experience these peaks and lows as uneven energy levels, one moment being wide awake and the next moment sleepy.

Eating little sugar and plenty of healthy fats and maintaining sufficient levels of minerals like chromium will keep your blood sugar and energy levels constant, without peaks and valleys. Our diet helps mother and baby to sidestep the disadvantages of sugar and carbs and to harness the long-lasting power of healthy fats, proteins, and minerals.

Sugar Hurts the Brain

The mother's sugar level has a big effect on how nerve cells are structured during early fetal development. High insulin levels from blood sugar spikes hurt the body's ability to form and nourish neurons. High insulin also inhibits synaptic transmission, in a sense muffling the communication between neurons. Too much sugar during pregnancy can spike your insulin levels and inhibit your baby's brain development.

Sugar and Carbohydrates Make Us Fat

In his book *Good Calories, Bad Calories: Fats, Carbs, and the Controversial Science of Diet and Health*, Gary Taubes argues against the idea that obesity is a matter of calories consumed and calories burned. Gary explains that excess sugar and carbohydrate intake is responsible for obesity because both of these substances boost insulin levels. High insulin levels are one reason people get fat, because insulin tells our bodies to store fat rather than burn it. When the insulin level is low, the body burns fat at a normal, consistent rate. Insulin regulates blood sugar by quickly transporting excess glucose into body cells, especially fat cells, which convert and store the energy from the glucose as fat.

From the perspective of epigenetics, sugar is almost certainly turning on bad genes that promote obesity in our kids. Mothers with either type 1 or type 2 diabetes are at a higher risk of having children who struggle with obesity. This is because the fetus is exposed to too much supplementary insulin. If a newborn is exposed to excess insulin, such as through mother's milk, this can also lead to childhood obesity.

Sugar Causes Infertility

Eating sugar makes it more difficult for a woman to conceive, because the ovaries are very sensitive to insulin, and because too much sugar turns off a gene that controls sex hormones. When the insulin level rises, insulin invades the hormone receptors on the ovaries that normally receive reproductive hormones. This disrupts the communication among the ovaries, the hypothalamus, and the pituitary glands, which can disrupt the female reproductive cycle. A high insulin level can also cause the ovaries to produce too many male sex hormones like testosterone, which disrupts the precise balance of the female reproductive system.

Sugar Promotes Oxidative Stress

High blood sugar or even a temporary spike in blood sugar causes oxidative stress in the body. Oxidative stress is a condition in which the body's ability to deal with toxins and repair the damage caused by them is compromised. This allows the toxins to cause more severe damage—perhaps permanent damage.

Fructose: The Worst Sugar of All

There's one kind of sugar that's more harmful than all the others: fructose. Fructose forms half of normal sucrose sugar molecules. Fructose is part of what makes sugar sweet, and it is the main sugar in fruit, which explains why we don't recommend eating a lot of fruit during pregnancy. The amount of fructose found in high-fructose corn syrup or agave syrup is much too high and has been associated with mineral depletion, high blood pressure, cardiovascular disease, miscarriage, and a decrease in sensitivity to insulin. Fructose also causes mineral imbalance and stimulates a process that accelerates aging. Fructose is low on the glycemic index (which measures the effects of foods on blood sugar and insulin), which is why products like agave syrup have been touted as health foods. Don't be fooled.

Small amounts of fructose (up to 25 grams per day) in the form of raw honey or fruit are safe and quite helpful for sleep when eaten in the evening.

Chemical Flavor Enhancers

There are many chemical flavor enhancers and sweeteners. The most common, however, are monosodium glutamate (MSG) and aspartame, and they pose the greatest risk.

MSG

Monosodium glutamate (MSG) is a chemical flavor enhancer that makes food seem like it tastes better than it really does. Glutamate is an excitatory neurotransmitter in the brain that is responsible for sending signals. In healthy brains, glutamate is sprayed into the synapses, the nerve fires, and then a reuptake process takes the glutamate back out of the synapse so the nerve stops firing.

Monosodium glutamate raises the glutamate level until the reuptake mechanism overloads. Upon overload, the glutamate sits in the synapse, which keeps the neuron firing over and over until it becomes exhausted or even dies. So MSG is a substance you'll want to keep away from your baby's brain. MSG is very common in Chinese and fast food, and it occurs naturally in soy sauce. For our guide to avoiding MSG, check out www.betterbabybook.com/msg.

Aspartame

Aspartame is an artificial chemical sweetener that is marketed as NutraSweet and Equal. It's sold under other names as well and is often used to sweeten diet soda. Aspartame is 40 percent aspartic acid (aspartate), an excitatory neurotransmitter that functions similarly to glutamate. Like glutamate, aspartate causes excess neuron firing and the eventual exhaustion and death of the neuron. Another 50 percent of aspartame is phenylalanine, which can build up in the body over time. Excess phenylalanine can enter the brain and lower the serotonin level, eventually resulting in emotional disorders or depression. The last 10 percent of aspartame is methanol, an alcohol that breaks down into two deadly poisons inside the body: formaldehyde and formic acid. Eighty-nine independent safety studies have found aspartame to be a health risk.

Aspartame is used heavily in processed food products, especially those labeled "diet," "sugar-free," and "no sugar added." It's also added to low-quality vitamin supplements and a host of medications. If a product contains aspartame, it will usually be on the ingredients list.

Other Chemical Flavor Enhancers

Other chemical sweeteners that have proven toxic effects inside the body are acesulfame K, saccharin, and sucralose (Splenda). They're found in many products similar to those that contain aspartame.

Most Grains

With the exception of rice, all grains including wheat, barley, oats, millet, rye, spelt, and quinoa contain antinutrients like phytic acid, and most of them contain glutenlike proteins that are bad news for a growing baby. Mycotoxins are also a real issue for many varieties of grain. Even just a little can have long-term effects on the health of your GI tract. For this reason, we recommend staying away from grains. Here are two of the most important ones to avoid.

Wheat

There are three reasons we avoided wheat during pregnancy and continue to avoid it now:

1. *Mycotoxins.* Wheat is easily contaminated with mycotoxins, especially in North America. Mold forms on the wheat when it's in the field and during processing and storage. Industrial farming has caused negative changes to soil ecology, which leads to more aggressive toxin-forming molds. Droughts or rain at the wrong time makes the problem even worse.

2. *Gluten.* Some people are sensitive to gluten and have major reactions to it (celiac disease), but beyond them, 80 percent of the world's population can't digest gluten effectively. In the gut, undigested gluten turns into a morphinelike compound called *gluteomorphin*, which has neurotoxic effects even on people

who aren't gluten-sensitive. We suspect this is why gluten-free diets seem to help with autism, which is a nerve-related disorder.

3. *Lectins.* Lectins are proteins found in a variety of foods. They're especially common in grains, beans, and seeds. Lectins have been linked to autoimmune inflammation and intestinal imbalance. Many food allergies are reactions to lectins.

The best thing you can do is to stop eating wheat (this includes bulghur and couscous), but if you still choose to, sprouted wheat is your best choice because lectins are destroyed when grains sprout. Wheat is so prevalent that it can be difficult to avoid. Nonetheless, removing it from our diet made us feel a lot better. We think it's a must.

If you do choose to eat unsprouted wheat, you can deal with the lectins by supplementing with N-acetyl-glucosamine and D-mannose (take them with the wheat). Lectins are more attracted to these sugar molecules than they are to others, so the sugars serve as effective decoys to bind any lectins in the gut and escort them out of the body.

Corn (Maize)

Corn is very susceptible to mycotoxins, and these days it's often genetically modified. Corn products are used in almost every processed food in supermarkets across the United States. The most common corn product you'll find is corn oil, one of the bad oils. This widespread use makes avoiding corn difficult.

Any animal that has eaten corn is just as unhealthy as the corn itself, and most farm animals are fed corn. This is one reason we recommend meat and butter from grass-fed cattle in the next chapter. Any product containing corn, any product refined from corn, and any product made from an animal that ate corn poses a high risk for exposing your baby to mycotoxins, the dangers of GMO foods, or excessive amounts of omega-6 fat and carbohydrates.

The only corn we eat is locally grown, organic, non-GMO corn on the cob in the summer. And even then, we eat it infrequently because it's so high in sugar.

Certain Legumes

Legumes, including soy, peanuts, and lentils, are not the health foods they've been made out to be. They are too high in sugar and carbohydrates and contain high amounts of antinutrients like phytic acid, and they tend to be very allergenic and difficult to digest. Traditional cultures used these foods only after a long period of soaking, sprouting, and fermentation. There is little benefit to adding these foods to your diet and some risk.

Soy

Even though a wide range of products made from soybeans have been marketed as a health food in recent years, research proves that (unfermented) soy is extremely unhealthy. Most soy products in the United States are not fermented. Unfermented soy is a problem for the following reasons:

1. It contains dangerous quantities of antinutrients, which are substances that block the body from absorbing important nutrients. The most notable are hemagglutinin, goitrogens, and phytic acid. Hemagglutinin promotes unhealthy blood clotting and blocks oxygen. Goitrogens prevent iodine from reaching the thyroid. Without iodine, the thyroid can enlarge and malfunction. Phytic acid blocks the body's absorption of essential minerals like calcium and magnesium.

2. It has lots of phytoestrogens, which do damage by mimicking estrogen inside the body.

3. It contains lysinoalanine, a known toxin, and nitrosamines, which are known carcinogens.

4. It has harmful levels of the mineral manganese and dangerous amounts of aluminum from being processed in aluminum containers.

5. It has a high risk of contamination with mycotoxins.

6. It is almost always genetically modified.

As you can see, soy has pretty much everything going against it. Fortunately, it's easy to avoid processed soy in the United States because it must be listed as an ingredient on product labels.

Most soy in Asian cuisine is different because it's been fermented. Fermentation greatly decreases the antinutrient and phytic acid levels. Fermented soy products include tempeh, miso, and natto. Most of these products are still highly processed and artificial, though, and soy sauce naturally contains MSG. To avoid GMO soy, make sure that any fermented soy product you eat is organic, or better yet just don't eat it at all.

Even in areas of the world like Asia where fermented soy is common, people actually don't eat much of it. A 1998 study found that Japanese men eat only about eight grams of soy per day (a teaspoon or two). The average misguided American consumes far more than this when he drinks a glass of soy milk or eats a soy burger (and these soy products aren't even fermented).

Peanuts

Peanuts are infamous for mold contamination, and that's why we avoid them. This contamination carries over into peanut butter and all other peanut products. Mycotoxins are probably why peanuts top the list of allergens in the United States. People have such violent reactions to peanuts that peanuts have been banned in many school lunchrooms. Given the peanut's susceptibility to mold, we're not surprised that traditional Chinese medicine includes peanuts in the *fa wu*, or toxic food, category. Peanuts are also high in omega-6 and won't help you lower your omega-6 to omega-3 ratio. Almond products are a great substitute for peanut products because they're delicious, they contain lower levels of omega-6, and they aren't as susceptible to molds.

Yeast

Saccharomyces cerevisiae—both baker's yeast and brewer's yeast—prevents the liver from detoxing your body as well as it can. It also helps harmful *Candida* yeasts grow, and it's atherogenic, which means it promotes the buildup of unhealthy cholesterol in the wrong places. Some misinformed people purposefully supplement with *S. cerevisiae*. Just because you see something at a health-food store doesn't mean it's healthy!

Mushrooms

Mushrooms are more mysterious and less well understood than many other organisms found in nature. We avoided mushrooms during pregnancy because people really don't know much about what they do inside the body. Different mushrooms produce such drastically different effects; some, considered "medicinal" mushrooms, do an excellent job of boosting the immune system and show great health benefits. Medicinal mushrooms usually grow on trees and include maitake, reishi, and shiitake.

Other mushrooms, like portobello mushrooms, taste good and appear to be harmless. Still others are hallucinogens, and some are deadly poisonous. We think it's okay to use medicinal mushrooms to build up immune support before pregnancy. However, we avoided all mushrooms during pregnancy because there are so many unknowns.

Pasteurized, Homogenized, or Conventional Dairy (Except Butter)

When we say *dairy*, we mean anything made from milk from cows, goats, and sheep, except butter. This includes milk, cheese (including cottage cheese and cream cheese), yogurt, sour cream, half and half, light cream, heavy cream, buttermilk, and ice cream. "Conventional" dairy is any dairy product that has not come from grass-fed, organically raised animals.

Pasteurization

The sale of raw dairy products is illegal in all states except California and Washington at the time of this writing because raw milk is, on rare occasions, contaminated with harmful pathogens that can compromise health. As a result, all dairy you'll find in any grocery store in the United States (except California and Washington) is pasteurized, or "cooked," dairy, including organic products from grass-fed cows.

Pasteurization, in which milk is heated to 150 degrees Fahrenheit for about thirty minutes and immediately stored at temperatures lower than 55 degrees Fahrenheit, is intended to reduce the risk of milk contamination substantially. But it also destroys most of the nutritional value of the milk, killing beneficial probiotics, denaturing (deforming) milk proteins, and transforming milk into an unhealthy substance that behaves like a clogging, irritating glue inside the body. The result is that what most Americans call "milk," and mistake for a healthy source of calcium and vitamin D, is actually linked to a host of health risks.

Pasteurization Destroys the Nutrients in Milk

Research has found that pasteurization reduces the vitamin content in milk, including vitamins C, A, and B complex. It transforms the lactose sugars found in milk into beta-lactose sugars, which are far more rapidly absorbed into the body. This rapid absorption causes sharper spikes in blood sugar and insulin and stronger swings in energy levels. Much of the calcium in pasteurized milk is useless to the human body; this might explain the observations in the mid-1930s that children fed raw milk had no tooth decay while children who drank pasteurized milk did have tooth decay. Pasteurization also destroys 20 percent of milk's natural iodine content. Considering that this has been known since the 1930s, it's a little surprising how few people know it.

Pasteurized Milk Can Cause Health Problems

The consumption of pasteurized milk has been linked to neurological disorders like autism. Casein, the primary protein found in milk, is permanently altered during the pasteurization process and becomes very difficult for the body to break down and digest. It is neurotoxic when present in high quantities.

Homogenization

Homogenization is a process that chemically alters milk so the cream no longer separates. Milk naturally contains xanthine oxidase (XO), a harmful enzyme involved in the production of uric acid that has been linked to oxidative stress. When nonhomogenized milk is consumed, the body is typically able to break down XO and prevent it from entering the bloodstream. Homogenized milk, however, contains XO that is surrounded with fat globules. In this form, XO makes its way into the bloodstream, and when this happens, it promotes cardiovascular disease.

Opium in Milk?

If you choose to consume raw milk products, be aware that the breed of cow is an important factor in milk selection. Milk from Holstein cows

("A1" cows) contains significant amounts of a dangerous protein called beta-casomorphin-7 (BCM-7), which is an opiate and can pose health risks. BCM-7 has been linked to autism, diabetes, and other diseases. Jersey, Asian, and African cows ("A2" cows) produce milk that contains only negligible amounts of BCM-7. It's entirely impractical to find this kind of milk since manufacturers don't tell you what cows made your milk, unless you're shopping at a small, local dairy. The vast majority of cows in the United States are A1-producting Holsteins.

If You Must Have Milk, Choose Organic Milk from Grass-Fed Cows

If you are simply unwilling to give up your dairy products during pregnancy, we strongly suggest that you find and use raw, organic milk products from grass-fed cows and consume them only when they're very fresh. If milk isn't from grass-fed cows, it's surely from grain-fed cows and thus poses all of the usual risks of grain. For example, mycotoxins are found in more than 10 percent of conventional creams. In the United States, milk that isn't organic usually comes from cows that were given recombinant bovine growth hormone, which has been linked to health problems, including cancer.

Is Milk Worth It These Days?

Because of the risk of contaminated raw milk and the health problems that pasteurized milk causes, we avoided dairy products during both pregnancies and continue to avoid them now. Our primary reason, aside from the research, is our own experience: we've enjoyed great health and have had wonderfully healthy babies without a drop of dairy products (except butter). Raw milk certainly has its health benefits, especially probiotics. But in the United States these days, raw milk is usually expensive (eight dollars per gallon is standard), it's hard to find, and it spoils quickly.

Why Is Butter Healthy, but Not Milk?

Milk proteins (including casein and BCM-7), which are the most harmful parts of milk, are present in butter only in very small quantities. What little milk protein remains in butter has been enzymatically modified during the butter fermentation process and isn't so unhealthy anymore. Dave is allergic to dairy protein but can eat butter without a problem. If people are sensitive to butter, they can often eat ghee. Butter is also low in mycotoxins—less than 2 percent of conventional butter is contaminated with mycotoxins. Some butters are much healthier than others. Organic butter from grass-fed cows is the healthiest. We cover it in the next chapter.

Cheese

Cheese is high in toxins and contains lots of denatured (cooked) casein, and some cheeses pose a risk of listeriosis. This is especially true of soft cheeses like brie, camembert, and feta; blue-vein cheeses such as Roquefort, Gorgonzola, and Stilton; and Mexican-style queso fresco, queso blanco, and panela.

All cheeses are made with yeast, other fungi, or bacteria, or all three. These organisms form toxins in the cheese that kill other organisms and prevent them from competing for the food source. These toxins also pose a threat to people. For instance, Roquefort cheese, made with the *Penicillium roqueforti* fungus, has a toxin in it called roqueforticin. Each brand of cheese and even each batch can have a different mix of fungi from the environment. This makes it very difficult to know if any particular cheese contains harmful amounts of toxins from bacteria or mycotoxins. Mycotoxins are found in more than 40 percent of conventionally produced cheeses.

Soft cheese and blue-vein cheeses are susceptible to contamination with *Listeria monocytogenes*, a harmful strain of bacteria found in water and soil. On occasion, *Listeria* is found in raw foods, especially raw meat and dairy products. Cooking or pasteurization kills *Listeria*. In the case of pasteurized soft and blue-vein cheeses, *Listeria* may actually be reintroduced between manufacturing and packaging. This is also a common threat with deli meats and reheated cooked foods, which we also discuss in this chapter.

Caffeine and Decaffeinated Products

There's lots of research showing that caffeine is unhealthy for mother and baby. When a pregnant woman consumes caffeine, even if not in excess, it has a noticeable effect on her fetus. Although an adult can break down caffeine rather quickly, a developing fetus has a much harder time. Since caffeine easily crosses the placenta, this means that caffeine easily builds up in the baby's body over time, even if the mother isn't consuming very much every day. Sustained exposure to excess caffeine can upset a fetus, raising the heart rate and causing squirming and discomfort in the womb. Caffeine also decreases blood flow to the placenta and causes the mother to absorb less iron and calcium from the foods she eats.

The risks of caffeine for a baby extend beyond pregnancy itself. It's suspected that women who consume more than 300 milligrams of caffeine (three cups of coffee) per day have more trouble conceiving. Caffeine also makes its way into breast milk and can cause the baby to become irritable and have trouble sleeping.

Decaffeinated coffee has also been linked to birth complications. We believe that mycotoxins are responsible. Coffee and tea (especially black tea) are commonly contaminated; one study found mycotoxins in more than 90 percent of tested coffee samples.

It turns out that caffeine is a natural antifungal. When caffeine is removed from coffee or tea, mold is able to grow more easily. Tests done on decaffeinated coffees found them to be much higher in mycotoxins. From this perspective, the Swiss Water Process of decaffeination isn't any safer—when it comes to avoiding mycotoxins, the removal of the caffeine *is* the problem!

How We Handled Caffeine during Pregnancy

While pregnant and nursing, Lana drank herbal teas, one cup of green tea per day, and allowed herself about half a cup of regular (not decaffeinated) coffee once every two weeks at most. When she did have coffee, it was made from high-end low-toxin cofee beans and prepared as espresso, because pressure and heat combined are known to destroy mycotoxins. Espresso preparation reduces the ochratoxin (a type of mycotoxin) level by more than 45 percent. Coffee is one of the most important things to buy organic, because conventional coffees are sprayed heavily with pesticides, and variations in processing matter. We use a special low-toxin coffee called upgraded coffee.

Garlic and Onions

Garlic and onions are known to desynchronize brain waves. A person's reaction time after eating garlic has been found to be two to three times slower than beforehand. For this reason, doctors recommend that pilots avoid garlic before flying. James Hardt, a psychologist who is a pioneer in EEG brain study, found that eating garlic and onions caused his study subjects to have lower levels of alpha brain waves. Alpha waves create the relaxed, alert, "in the zone" state that's associated with meditation and easy learning. In addition, a wide variety of Eastern medical traditions stress using garlic only for medicinal reasons, as regular use leads to anxiety.

Garlic does have health benefits; for example, it boosts immune function by killing unhealthy gastrointestinal microbes and is known to have cardiovascular benefits. Most of these benefits are available only in fresh raw garlic that has been finely chopped or crushed recently. This means that other forms of garlic—including dried, bottled, pickled, roasted, and in the form of supplements aren't very useful, yet they still contain neurotoxins.

We found it easy enough to get these benefits from other foods and avoid the neurotoxins at the same time. For example, vitamins D3 and C boost immune function, iodine combats infection, and ginger and hawthorn berry extract promote cardiovascular health.

Most Seafood

Before industrialization, fish was one of the healthiest things you could eat for your baby. Most fish is rich in protein, vitamin D, and omega-3. Because of modern pollution, however, most fish now contains dangerous levels of mercury.

Coal power plants across the United States expel about forty tons of mercury into the air every year. It settles on bodies of water and gets into the fish. If a pregnant woman eats even one serving of contaminated fish, her baby can suffer neurological damage. If you've eaten a lot of fish in the past, we recommend getting your mercury level measured and following our techniques for detoxing heavy metals (see chapter 13) before, not during, pregnancy.

Wild Caught Fish to Avoid

The FDA recommends avoiding shark, swordfish, tilefish, and king mackerel during pregnancy. Other studies have found unsafe levels of mercury in catfish, cod, crab, Great Lakes salmon, halibut, lake white-fish, largemouth bass, mahi mahi, marlin, pike, pollock, sea bass, tuna (steaks or canned), walleye, white croaker, and all shellfish (lobster, clams, oysters, mussels, squid, scallops, and shrimp). The studies also found mercury in the following species, though at a lower level: black or red grouper, bluefish, bonito, flounder, lake trout, orange roughy, perch, porgy, red snapper, rockfish, sole, and yellowtail.

The Truth about Farmed Fish

Like commercial beef, farm-raised fish is often raised on grain feed. This results in the omega-3 fatty acids becoming malformed and mostly devoid of benefit. Farm-raised fish are also fed conventionally grown grains that contain harmful pesticides and mycotoxins and might be GMOs. Farmed salmon in particular is fed soy and rendered poultry litter (that's used hen-house bedding, complete with chicken manure!), given high doses of pesticides and antibiotics, and dyed so it looks more pink.

Unless the package says "wild," a salmon product is probably farmed using these methods (note: "fresh" is not "wild"). Farmed GMO salmon is being considered for approval by the FDA, and even though there haven't been any studies done on the health effects yet, we'd certainly recommend avoiding it.

If you know a local fish farmer who raises fish the exact same way they grow in the wild, then farmed fish can be a good, mercury-free way to enjoy fish and get the health benefits. Unfortunately, we haven't yet found a fish farmer who does this.

Safe Fish

At the time of this writing, there are still several species of wild caught fish that aren't usually contaminated with mercury: flounder, haddock, Pacific sockeye salmon, Petrale sole, sardines, wild tilapia, and wild freshwater sport fish like trout. In the next chapter, we explain why these fish are your best choice.

Cured and Precooked Meats

Cured meats or any precooked meat, including deli meats and hot dogs, often contain nitrates or nitrites, which are preservatives that prevent oxidation (discoloration) of the meat. Sodium nitrate is most common. Nitrates themselves aren't too toxic, but when they're ingested, they convert to nitrites and disrupt cellular respiration (the ability of a cell to create energy).

Even if you find natural cured or precooked meats that are nitrate- and nitrite-free, these meats are among the highest-risk foods for *Listeria* contamination. Like cheeses, cured and precooked meat products often sit in display cases for a while, making most of them "old food" before you even buy them.

Certain Herbs

There are certain herbs that stimulate abnormal hormonal activity in the body. Some of them even stimulate and relax the uterus, which may cause premature birth. Here's a list of herbs to avoid during pregnancy: barberry, blue cohosh, celandine, dong quai, ephedra, ginseng, golden-seal, guarana, kola nut, passion flower, pau d'arco, pennyroyal, Roman chamomile, saw palmetto, and yohimbe.

Black cohosh is an herb that supports normal uterine function and menstrual cycles. We don't think it should be used during pregnancy without the oversight of a professional midwife, doctor, or health-care practitioner. The primary places to look out for these herbs are herbal teas and natural cosmetics. Beyond these sources, you probably won't come into contact with them.

Canned Food

The cans that are used to package foods contain a plastic resin lining that frequently contains bisphenol-A (BPA). Acidic canned foods, like toma-toes, are especially risky because the acidity encourages the BPA to leach into the food. Unless you're sure the resin lining is BPA-free, dehydrated or shrink-wrapped food or food in a jar is a safer way to consume preserved foods. Traditional canning in glass containers is a great way to preserve food, but like any hand-canned product, botulism is a risk to consider. Commercial canned foods often contain lots of preservatives as well.

Old Food

Ayurvedic tradition holds that eating old food, or "leftovers," creates poor digestion. We tested this idea by going a month without eating cooked leftovers. Of course, we avoided eating leftovers at home, but to avoid them completely we had to learn that old food is frequently disguised as fresh food, including anything in your local grocery store that is the following:

- Perishable
- Precooked
- Prepackaged cooked "fresh" food
- Unfrozen "ready to eat"
- "Fresh" deli-style meats, cheeses and other foods that sit in a display case

Leftovers also include almost all restaurant foods, which are usually precooked or prepared as much as several days in advance.

When our monthlong trial period was over, we definitely noticed better digestion and higher energy levels. Lana especially noticed higher energy during both pregnancies. We felt so much better that neither of us eats any old food anymore. Even when dealing with fresh food, we're more careful about how we store it. If it can be frozen, we freeze it and use it directly out of the freezer.

We suspect that old food is harmful because it's so easily contaminated with bacteria and mold. Although fresh food has some ability to resist bacterial and fungal colonies, once the food is cooked, that ability is lost. Cooking destroys most bacteria and mold spores, but when the food sits on the table, spores from the air recolonize it quickly. As soon as you put leftovers in the refrigerator, bacteria or fungi start growing again.

Making economical use of leftovers can be important in meeting a budget. Healthy food is expensive, and waste is waste—we're certainly not recommending that. Our solution was to practice cooking just the right amount of food so we didn't have leftovers or waste anymore. After a week or two, we got pretty good at it! If time constraints and budget won't allow for this and you must use leftovers, at least freeze them right away and heat them up without a microwave, directly out of the freezer.

Conventional Produce

Conventional produce (as opposed to organic produce) is fresh fruits and vegetables raised with pesticides, herbicides, and fungicides (farming chemicals). These toxic chemicals are sprayed on almost all conventional produce while it's growing. They help crops to grow and to avoid destruction from pests, predatory plants and weeds, and fungi and molds. Although it's great that these chemicals help crops to grow, unfortunately they stay in the produce permanently and pose a threat to people.

You can avoid most of these sprays by buying USDA organic produce, which is required to be free of pesticides, herbicides, and fungicides. The most heavily sprayed produce are apples, cantaloupe (Mexican), carrots, celery, cherries, coffee, cucumbers, grapes (imported), green and red bell peppers, green beans, kale, lettuce, nectarines, peaches, pears, spinach, and strawberries. By making sure you eat these products organic only, you can cut your exposure to farm chemicals by about 80 percent.

The following produce is generally safe to buy conventional: asparagus, avocados, bananas, broccoli, brussels sprouts, cabbage, cauliflower, eggplant, grapes (domestic), kiwi, mangoes, papaya, pineapple, plums, sweet potatoes, tomatoes, and watermelon. We think avocados are the safest conventional produce on the market.

Foods with Added Chemicals or Conditioners

Chemicals and conditioners are used in processed foods for countless reasons. So many unique agents are used that we'll just list the categories here: acidifiers, alkalizers, antibiotics, anticaking and antifoaming agents, bleaches, buffers, chemical (artificial) flavors, clarifiers, defoliants, deodorants, disinfectants, drugs, drying agents, dyes and colorings like cochineal or titanium dioxide, emulsifiers, expanders, high-fructose corn syrup, hydrolyzers, modifiers, moisteners, neutralizers, noxious sprays, stabilizers, steroids, synthetic hormones, synthetic vitamins that are barely usable by the body, and thickeners like carrageenan and propylene glycol. Not all of these additives are harmful, but studies have suggested that more than 90 percent of them are. If you see them on a product label, it's probably best to avoid the product.

Processed Foods

By "processed foods" we mean foods that for some reason aren't natural. Processed foods include the following:

- Genetically modified foods
- Foods containing hydrogenated oils (trans fat)
- Pasteurized or homogenized foods
- Prepared foods
- Crops grown with herbicides, pesticides, and fungicides
- Foods containing preservatives, artificial sweeteners (such as aspartame), or flavor enhancers (such as MSG)
- Foods containing a variety of chemical agents

Even though we detailed these topics earlier in the chapter, we find it helpful to group them together under "processed foods" because they're easier to remember that way.

5

Nourishing a Healthy Brain and Body

Thinking about changing your diet can be intimidating, but the payoff for eating a healthy, toxin-free diet is worth it. This chapter tells you how to do it.

The basis for a healthy diet is—yes!—fat. The belief that a low-fat diet is healthy is based on the assumption that all types of fat are the same, which is completely mistaken. The truth is that all fats are not created equal. There are good fats and bad fats, and in this chapter we will help you to distinguish between the two, which is important because pregnant women who try to minimize all fat in their diet do so at the risk of great harm to themselves and their babies.

Fat is one of the main building blocks of your body—and your baby's body. The body's brain, cell walls, and hormones are composed mostly of fat. Toxin-free healthy fats are some of the most nutrient-packed foods available; the issue is knowing where to find them. Your body metabolizes healthy fats more efficiently and with fewer waste products than either carbohydrates or proteins. Eating healthy fats keeps your baby's brain growing, gives you a feeling of satiety, and maintains your weight at optimal levels. If you make healthy fat a primary part of your diet, you actually *reduce* your risk of diabetes and heart disease.

Similarly, if you minimize your consumption of bad fats, you maximize your own health and increase your chances of giving birth to a vibrantly healthy baby with optimal brain development.

The research supporting a high-protein, healthy-fat diet goes back more than 150 years, and it took just 5 years to assemble it into more than 500 pages of plain English. We didn't have to do that, because Gary Taubes, the author of *Good Calories, Bad Calories*, already did. If our diet recommendations make you uncomfortable, you owe it to yourself—and your baby—to read his book. It supports our diet, which works for pregnant women, women seeking to get pregnant, and men working to build the healthiest sperm. And the basic principles apply to just about everybody at all stages of life. Here are some of the facts supporting our recommendations:

Facts about Fats

- The best fats are saturated and monounsaturated. Such fats are found in egg yolks, butter from grass-fed cows, coconut, meat from healthy grass-fed animals, avocados, olives, and nuts.

- Coconut oil is high in healthy saturated fats. These healthy fats optimize cholesterol levels, help our immune systems to fight intruders, contribute to healthy brain and hormone formation, and are an excellent source of energy.

- Omega-3 fatty acids, which are plentiful in wild caught salmon and the yolks of eggs from free-range hens, soothe the body by reducing inflammation, protecting us from exposure to too much omega-6, improving blood circulation, optimizing blood pressure, and healing scar tissue.

- Chemically processed omega-6 fatty acids are found in soy, canola, corn, and vegetable oils. Natural forms are found in nuts, vegetables, and grains. We need a small amount of omega-6, but this is overly abundant in the standard Western diet, which is rich in unhealthy oils and grains. In addition, omega-6 oxidizes easily, which makes eating it especially unhealthy when it's cooked.

- Fats that are oxidized, hydrogenated (trans fat), or contaminated by mycotoxins—including many of the fats used in processed food, margarine, and so-called butter spreads and substitutes—can cause heart disease, high blood pressure, and diabetes. In the previous chapter, you learned how to avoid these fats. Our diet includes none of them.

Facts about Carbohydrates

- Carbohydrates in the form of fructose (fruit sugar), refined or whole grains, and other starches make you hungry, slow your metabolism so that you burn fewer calories, and lower your physical activity levels. They do the same for your fetus.

- Carbohydrates contribute to obesity (and later heart disease) because they lower insulin sensitivity, which results in a higher overall insulin level and a tendency to store fat. When insulin sensitivity gets very low, it's called insulin resistance, which is one step away from type 2 diabetes. Pregnant women need to be particularly concerned about high insulin levels because they may lead to a dangerous condition called pregnancy-related diabetes.

- Conventional advice tells us to eat fruit and vegetables, always mentioning the two in one breath as though they are equally beneficial, but the truth is that fruits contain different types and amounts of sugar than vegetables do. The type of sugar in fruit (fructose) lowers insulin sensitivity and raises some risk factors for heart disease (like triglycerides), whereas the type of sugar in vegetables (glucose) does not.

- Exercise causes weight loss not so much because it burns calories but primarily because it increases insulin sensitivity. Higher insulin sensitivity means a lower overall insulin level, and less insulin means less fat storage.

The Food Pyramid

This is what the famous food pyramid should really look like:

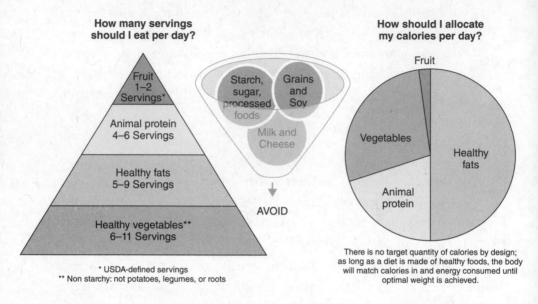

How many servings should I eat per day?

Fruit
1–2
Servings*

Animal protein
4–6 Servings

Healthy fats
5–9 Servings

Healthy vegetables**
6–11 Servings

Starch, sugar, processed foods

Grains and Soy

Milk and Cheese

↓

AVOID

* USDA-defined servings
** Non starchy: not potatoes, legumes, or roots

How should I allocate my calories per day?

Fruit

Vegetables

Animal protein

Healthy fats

There is no target quantity of calories by design; as long as a diet is made of healthy foods, the body will match calories in and energy consumed until optimal weight is achieved.

When we described our diet to friends who were also expectant mothers, we often heard two things. First they would exclaim, "Fat! Are you sure? I gained thirty-five pounds with my first baby, and I still haven't lost the last ten pounds!" Or if this was her first pregnancy, the woman always had a sister, a friend, or a colleague who was still battling the baby weight, months and even years later. Fat was the last thing she was going to put on her plate. After the initial disbelief, the second question was "If I shouldn't eat grains, legumes, processed foods, or even very much fruit, what am I supposed to eat?"

That's why this book uses both a food pyramid and a pie chart. The food pyramid shows the number of daily servings we recommend of various foods, and the pie chart shows the percentage of total daily calories those foods should constitute. The pie chart shows us that fat, being a very calorie-dense food, should make up the largest percentage of calories in your diet. The pyramid shows us that vegetables, being composed mostly of water and containing relatively few calories, should make up the largest number of servings in your diet. You have to eat a lot of them to get the nutrients they offer, which are different nutrients from those found in meat.

In this chapter, we identify the healthiest foods you can find—the foods that should be the cornerstones of your lifelong diet even if you're not planning a pregnancy. For each food, we detail why our recommendation makes sense, offer tips about the healthiest ways to prepare it, and tell you how to work it into your routine. If you're already convinced, go to the end of this chapter to find the diagrams listing these healthy foods.

Eggs

Organic eggs from free-range hens are loaded with valuable nutrients, and Lana ate countless eggs during both pregnancies. Tryptophan, selenium, iodine, phosphorus, riboflavin, choline, folate, lutein, zeaxanthin, vitamin D, and lots of good protein and fats are just a few of the reasons to eat healthy eggs. Most of the nutrients in the egg are in the yolk, along with half of the protein and all of the healthy fat.

One egg contains six grams of protein—three in the yolk and three in the white. This protein is of excellent quality because it contains all of the essential amino acids, distributed in almost perfect proportions. Eggs help young adults to construct stronger muscles and older adults to prevent muscle loss. The protein in properly prepared eggs is wonderful raw material that supports a baby's growth. Eggs support eye health because they contain forms of lutein that are very bioavailable. Eggs are also high in B vitamins, a class of vitamins that plays a big role in the development of a baby's nervous system. Finally, eggs are rich in iron, which guards against anemia.

In terms of pregnancy, perhaps the most important thing about eggs is the choline found in the yolk. Choline is an essential nutrient that is known to be an integral part of a baby's brain development. It also guards against birth defects. The National Academy of Sciences suggests 450 milligrams of choline per day for pregnant women and 550 milligrams per day for breast-feeding mothers. A pregnant woman can get almost half of the minimum daily choline she needs—250 milligrams—from two eggs, but we recommend exceeding minimum recommendations by a large margin because our goal is to optimize health, not simply to prevent malnutrition. Eggs aren't our only source of choline (so you don't need to eat four or more eggs every day), but they're a great source.

It turns out that choline is beneficial for everyone. In adults, choline is key to cell function (especially neural function), liver metabolism, and disease prevention. For example, a 2008 study linked high choline intake with a 24 percent lower rate of breast cancer. Women over nineteen need 425 milligrams every day, and men over nineteen need 550 milligrams. Research has found that only one in ten Americans gets enough choline every day.

Many people believe that eggs are unhealthy because they are high in cholesterol, but the facts suggest otherwise. There is cholesterol in eggs, but eating it won't harm you unless you oxidize it by overcooking it. That's why we recommend eating yolks soft-cooked or raw but not hard-cooked. A 2006 study in Britain found that eggs have not been linked with heart disease. In 2007, another study found that ninety-five hundred people eating one or more eggs every day did not experience a greater rate of heart disease or stroke. The study also found that eating eggs actually decreased blood pressure. Yet another study, also from 2007, concluded that recommendations to limit egg intake were not based on scientific evidence. It seems that "eggs are bad" is one of those myths based on questionable science from decades ago, but one that refuses to die.

Eating eggs will also help you to avoid excess weight gain before, during, and after pregnancy. Eggs contain a great balance of healthy fat and protein, so eating them helps you to feel both energized and satisfied. The more satisfied you feel, the less you'll be tempted to snack on empty calories like carbohydrates.

There is little or no downside to adding eggs to a Better Baby diet, but there is a significant upside.

Healthy Hens Make Healthy Eggs

As healthy as good eggs are, some eggs are much better for you than others, for all eggs are not created equal. Hens, just like humans, can produce healthy eggs only if their diet and environment are healthy. This means that they are able to graze outside in an organic field. As our local egg seller says, "They eat what they can find: bugs, grasses, seeds, and worms." The nutrients from pasture grasses, bugs, and sun exposure make the eggs much healthier than commercial eggs from hens raised in confinement, fed poor-quality feed, and deprived of sun exposure.

Experiments done in 1933 found that chickens fed only soy, corn, wheat, or cottonseed meal didn't even lay eggs. They were simply not healthy enough. If, however, they were permitted access to fresh pasture grass and bugs in addition to the feed, they started laying eggs again. The nutrients in the pasture grass and bugs are essential.

Later studies found that eggs from free-range hens are richer in a variety of nutrients than those from factory-farmed hens. In 1974, a British study discovered that free-range eggs were much higher in folate and vitamin B12. In 1998, researchers discovered that free-range eggs have 30 percent more vitamin E than commercial eggs do. And, in 2007, *Mother Earth News* published a study it conducted comparing the nutrient content of eggs sampled from fourteen free-range farms across the United States with the nutrient content of eggs from hens raised in confinement. The findings were impressive. The free-range eggs contained 66 percent more vitamin A, twice the amount of omega-3 fatty acids, and a remarkable seven times more beta-carotene.

Free-range eggs are pretty easy to find these days, so we strongly recommend buying them to give yourself and your baby all these extra health benefits. They also taste better! Sadly, "free range" from stores usually come from chickens that did not actually have access to outdoor organic pastures to feed on their natural diet of grasses and bugs. "Cage-free" eggs can come from birds raised indoors, in overcrowded conditions and without access to the outdoors. The yolks of free-range eggs will typically be a much richer, deeper yellow than the yolks of commercial eggs. When deeper color is natural in a food, it's often an indication of high nutrient content.

Egg Warnings

Sulmonella contamination of eggs is all over the news these days. In 2010, half a billion eggs from Iowa were recalled. Knowing the health benefits of eggs, we decided to look at the risks versus the rewards, and we're convinced that the benefits of eating raw egg yolks far outweigh the risk of *Salmonella*, especially if you take the simple precautions we describe here.

The rate of *Salmonella* contamination in eggs is about one in twenty thousand. That's incredibly low. This is an average for all eggs, including commercially raised factory-farm eggs, which make up the vast majority of what's on the market. The organic free-range eggs we recommend are safer because the organic environment produces healthier chickens that better resist disease and infection. Most of the time, *Salmonella* is not going to be on healthy eggs that were properly refrigerated. And if it is, it's likely to be on the shell and not inside the egg unless the shell is cracked. In that case, any *Salmonella* that was present on the outside of the shell will infect the inside of the egg. For this reason, we never eat eggs that have been cracked, even if the crack is slight. We urge any pregnant woman to use the same caution and recommend you wash your eggs before cracking them.

Preparing Safe Eggs

How eggs are cooked determines how healthy they'll be. If the yolks are overcooked, most of the healthy nutrients will be altered in such a way that they no longer optimize health. In fact, the oxidized cholesterol from hard-cooked yolks is actively unhealthy.

Overcooked egg whites—whites cooked to the point of being crisp or browned at the edges—aren't healthy, because they're oxidized. Conversely, if you eat too many egg whites that are raw, especially if you eat them without the yolk, you may develop a deficiency of a B vitamin called biotin, which is important in blood sugar regulation and hair and nail growth.

The perfectly prepared egg has lightly cooked whites and a runny yolk. But keep in mind that perfection is not our goal. Moving *toward* perfection is our much more achievable goal, and you're better off eating almost any egg cooked any way you like, as long as the yolk isn't overcooked. Hard-boiled or overcooked scrambled eggs are not healthy.

When we eat eggs raw, we gently wash the shells with a mixture of a few drops of iodine or grapefruit seed extract (GSE, available at most health food stores) in a bowl of water before opening them. And if we're feeling particularly concerned about the safety of an egg, we may even put a drop of edible GSE on the yolk after opening the egg, just to make sure to kill all the harmful microbes, including *Salmonella*. If we don't have those substances handy, we just use hot water and dishwashing liquid to wash the shell. Washing or sterilizing eggs before opening them reduces the risk of a *Salmonella* infection nearly to zero. During the wash, we submerge the eggs in water. If we see a thin stream of bubbles, that means the shell is cracked, and even if we can't see the crack, we don't eat the egg.

After washing the eggs, we use them in one of several ways. Often we simply add the raw yolks to our smoothies. If we cook the eggs, we put them in a frying pan with lots of butter (from grass-fed cows) on very low heat until the egg white is soft but solid. It should be completely white. If any of the egg white on top is still runny, we use a culinary torch (widely available at cookware stores and by mail order) to cook it, making sure we leave the yolk raw. This makes for great sunny-side up eggs that aren't burned on the bottom and that therefore don't contain harmful free radicals in blackened, oxidized parts. It is interesting to note that this technique is widely used to make perfect eggs at leading gourmet restaurants around the country. As an alternative, you can just flip the egg over very briefly until the white solidifies but the yolk is still soft and runny.

Lana ate lots of eggs—more than two or three per day—during both pregnancies and while nursing. Not only did Lana have healthy pregnancies, her blood fat and cholesterol levels are perfect.

Coconut

When we suggest to mothers that they should eat coconut, the most common response we hear is "But isn't coconut full of cholesterol?" The answer is no. Coconut oil is high in healthy saturated fat but has no cholesterol. The popular belief that coconuts are unhealthy was manufactured in the mid-1980s by the American Soy Association, which created a propaganda campaign against coconut oil in order to enrich U.S. soy farmers.

Throughout history, many different cultures have valued coconut highly as both a food and a medicine. Modern science has discovered many of the reasons. According to the Coconut Research Center in Colorado Springs, coconut can kill bacteria as well as viruses, fungi, and parasites. People who live in the Pacific Islands and parts of Asia where a lot of coconut is consumed have lower rates of cardiovascular disease, cancers, and other degenerative diseases associated with the Western diet.

A 1960s study examined the populations of two Pacific islands— Pukapuka and Tokelau—that totaled about twenty-five hundred people. The Polynesian people, who are the main inhabitants of these islands, have adhered to their traditional ways of living, including their diet, which is high in saturated fat from coconut, high in fiber, and low in sugar. The people were lean and healthy—much more so than their Western counterparts—and had very low rates of disease.

The study noted that when some of the Polynesian people migrated to New Zealand and switched to eating a Western-type diet, they experienced higher cholesterol and an increased rate of cardiovascular disease. The point is that people who eat coconut instead of other fat sources (typically high in unhealthy polyunsaturated and hydrogenated fats) are far healthier than people who don't.

For a long time, people in the United States and Europe believed that coconut is unhealthy because of its saturated fat content. We now know that the opposite is true. The fats in coconut are mostly medium-chain triglycerides (MCTs). It's the MCT content that makes coconut such a powerful antibiotic, viricide, fungicide, and parasiticide. MCTs also promote a healthy cholesterol level and help to prevent heart disease. Maybe that's why people in Panama have been known to drink coconut oil by the glass to fight illness. It's certainly why we use both coconut oil and MCT oil, a coconut oil extract that further boosts the number of energizing MCTs in our diet.

Unlike the MCTs in coconut, almost all other fats in our diet, from animals and plants alike, are long-chain fatty acids. Because the length of a fatty acid makes a big difference in how it will be used inside the body, the fact that coconuts are the only food we eat that has a significant number of MCTs gives it a particularly important role in our health.

Coconut oil is a source of many of the various types of healthy fats your body needs to make a healthy baby, and each fat has unique benefits. Half of coconut oil is lauric acid, one of the components of breast milk that helps to fight bacteria. Coconut also contains two other healthy fats, caprylic acid and capric acid, which are available as energy immediately after you eat them with no extra processing by your body. For a healthier pregnancy and for the best breast milk, you should get plenty of these three kinds of fat in your diet. The best way to do that is to consume coconut oil, using it to cook with or in various dressings and sauces.

You should add MCT oil to your diet, too. MCT oil is not a replacement for coconut oil, because it lacks lauric acid, but we particularly like it because it provides a noticeable energy boost and because, being flavorless, it's very versatile in its uses.

Coconut oil kills more than twenty-five viruses, bacteria, and other microorganisms that cause a number of ailments, including ulcers, throat and urinary tract infections, gum disease and cavities, pneumonia, and gonorrhea. Coconut oil has a devastating effect on yeasts like *Candida*, which is why Polynesian women almost never experience yeast infections. Coconut oil also kills or weakens a number of parasites and worms, including giardia, tapeworm, and lice. To prevent disease and infection, you just can't go wrong with coconut oil. Despite its powerful antibiotic properties, however, coconut oil doesn't harm the probiotic flora population in your gastrointestinal tract.

Two of the most important times for a woman to consume coconut oil are while she's pregnant and when she's lactating, because coconut oil raises the levels of important fatty acids present in the mother's milk to their highest levels, serving as perfect food for growth and as initial immune protection for her baby.

Eating coconut oil will also give you beautiful skin and shiny hair. It's a great source of energy and will help you to stay awake and alert throughout the day. It boosts fat metabolism and promotes weight control.

Lana ate coconut in some form—oil, MCT oil, or fresh young coconuts—nearly every day while pregnant or nursing. The results were very noticeable, especially in her skin and hair. In fact, her hair stylist was blown away when she saw the positive changes in Lana from the diet. She said that in her experience, the later stage of pregnancy and nursing "wrecks women's hair and skin" and couldn't believe that Lana had been nursing Anna for almost a year. When the stylist asked Lana what brand of skin-care products she was using, she was even more surprised to hear Lana say, "Food. I don't need anything else."

Both plain coconut oil and MCT oil are great for cooking, because unlike many cooking oils used today, they are fully saturated and therefore don't oxidize at normal cooking temperatures. This makes for a diet that will produce fewer cancer-causing free radicals throughout the body. Both coconut oil and MCT oil are very stable in heat, so they're safe for gentle cooking (not frying).

In terms of dietary requirements, coconut oil is almost a complete fat by itself, but it doesn't contain omega-3. Since the body needs omega-3 to survive, it's important to realize that coconut oil is not enough by itself. No single fat source is likely to contain all of the kinds of fat the body needs. By mixing sources, however, you can cover all of the bases and achieve optimal health. Eating coconut oil along with avocados, beef and lamb from grass-fed animals, butter from grass-fed cows, raw egg yolks, and wild caught sockeye salmon, and perhaps supplementing with fish oil as well, will certainly do the trick.

When introducing coconut oil (or any oil) into your diet, be careful not to add too much over too short a period, or you may experience indigestion, intestinal cramping, or diarrhea. Teach your body how to use fat for fuel by starting slowly, such as by adding just one tablespoon of coconut oil or MCT oil to two of your daily meals for two or three days. Then, over the course of the next two weeks or so, gradually increase to a total of four to six tablespoons per day or more, spread across all of the day's meals, if you can tolerate it.

If you experience any of the symptoms described above, just drop down to a level that you tolerated well, and try to increase again a few days later. Besides cooking with coconut oil and adding it to our salads, smoothies, and recipes, we each eat about four to six tablespoons of coconut oil per day. This is in addition to the other healthy oils we've discussed.

Coconut Tips: How to Buy and Cook with Coconut Products

There are a few things to remember about buying and eating coconut. You can't go wrong buying fresh organic young coconuts in the produce section (the white-husked ones, not the brown ones). If you're not eating raw coconut, keep in mind that many processed commercial coconut products are likely to contain large amounts of refined sugar, so stay away from these. Organic dried shredded coconut is a fine choice if it doesn't contain extra sugar.

When buying coconut oil, choose either organic cold-processed or expeller-pressed. These forms of processing preserve the most MCTs and are truest to the coconut's original (and healthiest) makeup. Cold-processed coconut oil carries a strong coconut flavor that complements some dishes, whereas expeller-pressed coconut oil has very little flavor.

MCT oil is liquid at room temperature and has no flavor, making it the perfect oil for light salad dressings or for coating vegetables. It also mixes into smoothies simply and quickly. Up-to-date information on where to buy high-quality, mycotoxin-free coconut oil and MCT oil is available on our website, www .betterbabybook.com/met.

Olives and Olive Oil

Olives and olive oil are a great source of monounsaturated fats, which optimize cholesterol levels and lower the risk of heart disease. The good form of cholesterol, HDL, is necessary to make the hormones in your body and in your baby's body. It's also necessary for the formation of your baby's brain and nervous system (starting in the womb) and for healthy brain function. According to Iowa State biophysics professor Yeon-Kyun Shin, if you deprive the brain of cholesterol, "then you directly affect the machinery that triggers the release of neurotransmitters. Neurotransmitters are involved in the data-processing and memory functions. In other words—how smart you are and how well you remember things."

Olive oil is a great source of powerful antioxidants and anti-inflammatory agents called *polyphenols*. Polyphenols play a key role in olive oil's ability to improve cardiovascular health and optimize cholesterol levels. Olive oil also reduces the risk of colon cancer and slows cognitive decline. Women in ancient Rome even applied olive oil externally to prevent stretch marks during pregnancy.

Olives themselves are a healthy food. They are great as an appetizer or used in almost any way you can imagine. We like to mix them into our burgers and salads. Green and black are both fine, as long as they are packed in real olive oil or are brine cured. Be aware, however, that most gourmet olives are packed in unhealthy soybean or canola oil, wine vinegar (which may be contaminated by mycotoxins), or other undesirable preservatives.

When choosing olive oil, choose organic extra-virgin olive oil, because it contains more polyphenols than the other two types of olive oil you commonly see, which are plain (not extra-) virgin, and light. Both virgin and light contain fewer polyphenols than extra-virgin olive oil does. That's why extra-virgin olive oil is more effective than lower grades of olive oil at optimizing cholesterol level.

Olive Oil Tips: Dress but Don't Cook with Olive Oil

Exposure to light and heat in storage will oxidize olive oil a little bit and detract from its health value, but cooking with olive oil makes it actively unhealthy. Heating olive oil for cooking has a pervasive oxidative effect, transforming it from a healthy oil into a free radical–generating oil worthy of a fast-food restaurant. This is true even when you lightly sauté vegetables in olive oil. There's no reason to ruin a perfectly good oil by doing that. We use olive oil all the time, usually as part of a salad dressing, but if we want it on hot food, we add it *after* the food has been cooked and is on our plates. And our young children love eating whole olives—both green and kalamata—as much as we do.

Like any oil that is not saturated, olive oil will oxidize and become rancid when it is exposed to too much light and heat. So when shopping for it, make sure that it is kept in a cool area and packaged in a tinted bottle for protection from light. And as with any food, glass containers are better than cans. Olive oil should always be consumed within a year of purchase, because after that time the phenol level as well as the carotenoid and chlorophyll levels drop, causing the oil to lose much of its health value. This will happen even if it's stored in your refrigerator.

Meat and Butter from Grass-Fed Animals

If this book hasn't already shocked you with science-backed advice that contradicts the conventional wisdom, get ready, because we are about to present the facts that fly in the face of the largest piece of nutritional dogma of all. We might as well start by just stating the truth: red meat and butter are some of the healthiest things you can eat—as long as they come from healthy animals.

No matter how much evidence supports this, and despite the thousands of years that people have eaten red meat, most people who hear this statement respond with disbelief, denial, disgust, or even anger. After all, if this is true (and it is), the guilt you felt every time you enjoyed steak was for nothing, and that flavorless butter substitute you smeared on your toast wasn't healthier (actually, it was unhealthy, but that's another story). Worst of all, it means you have been lied to about your health, and the people who were supposed to be keeping you safe were asleep on the job.

That's how we felt when we did the research and switched to meat and butter from grass-fed animals. In fact, all of the people we've counseled, pregnant or not, who have followed our advice to increase their intake of healthy beef, lamb, and butter reported large increases in energy and mental clarity, easy muscle formation, and fat loss, usually within two to four weeks. Lana ate red meat and multiple tablespoons of butter nearly every day during both pregnancies. Both of us *felt* healthier from eating butter and meat, and the profound improvements in our lipid chemistry (a summary of the levels of HDL, LDL, triglycerides, and other fats in the bloodstream) showed that we actually *were* healthier.

The reason for these changes is that we were cutting polyunsaturated oils from our diet and replacing them with more stable, health-enhancing saturated and monounsaturated fats.

We'll be the first to tell you, however, that all meat and butter are not created equal, and we consciously chose the right sources. If you decide to increase your intake of meat and dairy to support your pregnancy, it's absolutely critical that you choose products from grass-fed animals. We'll go into a little detail to make the case that switching to meat and butter from grass-fed animals will have a huge impact on your health—and your baby's, too.

Good Meat, Bad Meat: Choose Beef and Lamb from Grass-Fed Animals

Meat from grain-fed cattle, sheep, or bison contains seven to eight grams of fat per three-ounce serving. That's about three times the fat content of meat from grass-fed animals, which averages two and a half grams per three-ounce serving. Meat from grass-fed animals is so low in fat that it's actually too low to support optimal hormone production for a pregnant woman. That's why it's a good idea to accompany a dish of this meat with a nice butter sauce or some guacamole.

But it's not just the amount of fat that matters, it's the type. Most of the fat in meat from grain-fed animals is easily oxidized polyunsaturated omega-6 fat. The fat in this meat also contains the unhealthy hormones that ranchers add to make the animal grow more quickly, along with mold toxins from poor-quality feed.

The fat that is in meat from grass-fed animals, in contrast, is almost entirely saturated and monounsaturated. It's actually healthy fat, which will support your baby's growing nervous system. A study published in the June 2008 *Journal of Agriculture and Food Chemistry* showed that the fat composition of meat from grass-fed animals is "clearly superior" to that of meat from grain-fed animals and "remarkably beneficial" for the human diet. Beef from grass-fed cattle has actually been shown to lower problem cholesterol levels.

How You Cook It Matters
Cook your meat to no more than medium, and instead of searing the outside, put the grill or oven at 250 to 300 degrees Fahrenheit and cook

the meat gently so it is not charred on the outside and is still pink inside. Use a digital meat thermometer if you need it. We cook our meat at a low temperature until the inside is 115 to 118 degrees Fahrenheit, then take it out of the oven. The meat continues to cook after it's removed; the internal temperature may rise another five degrees before we serve it.

Even healthy fats can be oxidized if they're cooked for too long or at too high heat. The different fat composition of meat from grass-fed animals makes them cook more quickly than meat from grain-fed animals. Always cook slowly and gently on low heat, whether you're cooking on the stove, on the grill, or in the oven.

The Benefits of Meat from Grass-Fed Animals

Meat from grass-fed cattle has two to four times more omega-3 fatty acids than meat from grain-fed animals does. That's because omega-3 is produced in the chloroplasts (the site of photosynthesis) of green leaves, including grass, and grass-fed cattle get to eat lots of them. The *Journal of Animal Science* published a study that tracked the omega-3 levels in grass-fed cattle that were switched to a grain-fed diet; the omega-3 levels decreased every day. The result was the same for the meat and eggs of chickens that have no access to fresh green foods.

Omega-3 is central to cell function and heart health. People who eat a diet rich in omega-3 experience lower rates of heart attack, depression, schizophrenia, ADHD, and Alzheimer's disease. Omega-3 has also been shown to slow the growth of some types of cancer. Nearly 20 percent of Americans have omega-3 blood levels that are so low they cannot be detected.

Meat from grain-fed animals also has a dangerously lopsided ratio of omega-6 to omega-3 fatty acids: fourteen to one! A high ratio of omega-6 to omega-3 fatty acids in the body has been linked to a variety of health problems, including increased rates of cancer and cardiovascular disease, among others. Four to one is a healthy dietary ratio of omega-6 to omega-3. The ratio in beef from grass-fed cattle is an even more optimal ratio of two to one, on par with most fish, including wild caught salmon.

Meat from grass-fed animals has also been shown to be three to five times higher than meat from grain-fed animals in conjugated linoleic acid (CLA), which reduces cancer tumor growth, increases lean body

Meat-Buying Tips

When purchasing meat from grass-fed animals, organic is best. But many "organic" meat products are not from grass-fed animals, so it's important to check that what you buy is *both* grass-fed and organic. If you can have only one, choose grass-fed over organic.

You should also be aware that some meat markets will advertise meat as being from grass-fed cattle when in fact the ranchers "grain-finish" the beef by feeding it grain for a month before slaughter. In other words, the animal was grass-fed, but then it was grain-fed, and the advertisers didn't feel the need to mention that detail. Although they aren't lying (they're technically correct—the cattle ate grass), meat from grain-finished cattle is less healthy than meat from cattle that were fully grass-fed. Don't be afraid to ask; in this case, it pays to know exactly what you're buying. The more grain a cow ate, the unhealthier its meat will be.

mass, and promotes healthy cardiovascular function. The same goes for vitamins A and E: meat from grass-fed cattle has two to four times as much of these important vitamins as meat from grain-fed cattle. It is also interesting to note that the meat from grass-fed cattle contained twice as much vitamin E as the meat from grain-fed cattle even when the grain-fed cattle were heavily supplemented with synthetic vitamin E.

Grain-fed cattle are far more susceptible than grass-fed cattle to infection with *E. coli* bacteria, which can be deadly to humans. The reduction in risk from aggressive *E. coli* species alone justifies the switch to meat from grass-fed animals.

What about Pork and Fowl?

It's true that if pigs, chickens, turkeys, ducks, and geese eat what they're supposed to, their meat will be healthier, too. But even when these animals eat a natural diet, their fats still aren't as healthy as beef and lamb from grass-fed animals. That's because they contain much more

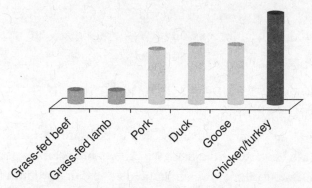

The amount of unhealthy polyunsaturated fat in animals

polyunsaturated fat than beef and lamb do. Polyunsaturated fats oxidize easily when they're cooked (or even exposed to oxygen or light) and become carcinogenic. Unfortunately, unlike beef and lamb, which can be eaten rare or medium rare, pork and fowl all must be cooked thoroughly to be eaten safely. So it's impossible to avoid oxidized polyunsaturated fats when eating these meats.

The fat from chicken and turkey is about 20 percent polyunsaturated, and the fat from duck and goose about 13 percent. That's a lot more polyunsaturated fat than in beef and lamb, which are only 3 percent, or in pork, which is 12 percent. This means that on average, eating pork is healthier than eating chicken or turkey. And, in fact, we do enjoy bacon for breakfast sometimes, provided it's cooked gently (thoroughly, but not charred or crispy).

You might look at the fat composition of olive oil, see that it's about 10 percent polyunsaturated fat, and wonder why we recommend eating that but not chicken, fowl, or pork. The trick is that we only eat olive oil that has not been used in cooking or otherwise heated. When polyunsaturated fats aren't heated and oxidized, a moderate amount is fine to eat.

If you do choose to eat fowl and pork, it's still important to buy products made from healthy animals that ate good-quality diets. For chicken and turkey, organic free-range is best. Duck and goose is by far the healthiest, if it's wild game. In the store, organic is best. As for pork, it's essential to find out what the pigs were fed. In the wild, pigs are omnivores and will forage for a variety of things. They'll eat vegetation, grass, roots, and any animal carcasses they find, including mice, rats, and rabbits. When raised domestically, pigs that were fed vegetables, roots, and protein feeds will typically produce healthier pork. Pork from pigs that were factory-farmed or that didn't eat natural foods isn't likely to be healthy.

Good Dairy, Bad Dairy: Choose Butter from Grass-Fed Animals

You know from chapter 4 that we don't recommend drinking milk or eating cheese because of the negative effects of casein, especially when the milk is pasteurized. However, butter is one dairy product that doesn't have much casein at all, and it's a healthy, satisfying part of our diet. Another reason to eat butter is that it's one of the oils you should use for cooking. It doesn't oxidize easily when heated.

When buying butter, it's just as important to choose butter made from grass-fed cows or goats as it is to choose meat made that way. The fat in butter from grass-fed cows is actually good for you, unlike the fat in butter made from grain-fed cows (and unlike what you have probably been led to believe).

Unfortunately, modern dairy practice confines cows and feeds them a diet high in grain, corn, and soy, which are not natural food sources for cattle. The reason for this strange diet is simple: it makes cows produce many more gallons of milk per day. In 1999, however, researchers discovered that the less milk a cow produces, the higher the concentration of vitamins and nutrients in the milk. In other words, a cow transfers the same amount of vitamins into her milk no matter how much milk she produces. Today's supercows may produce twenty times as much milk, but their milk is severely diluted in terms of its vitamin content.

A look at other research shows that many of the benefits of meat from grass-fed animals are also found in butter from grass-fed animals. A 2006 study concluded that the more that fresh pasture was added to a cow's diet, the more omega-3 the butter contained. Butter from grass-fed cows contains far more vitamins E and A, beta-carotene, and CLA than butter from grain-fed cows. Butter concentrates the fat-soluble nutrients from milk, but only if the nutrients are present in the first place, of course. Grass-fed cows' butter is lower in mycotoxins, both because there's less mold on grass than on grains and because milk processing concentrates the toxins in the milk solids, most of which are removed when making butter.

Butter-Buying Tips

Some specialty markets sell butter from grass-fed cows, but it's expensive. A better way to get it is to buy butter from Ireland and New Zealand, since in these countries it's cheaper to feed a cow grass than grain. We maintain a list of grass-fed brands at www .betterbabybook.com/butter.

Also keep in mind that *organic* is not the same as *grass-fed*. Organic butter costs more because the ranchers feed organic corn, wheat, and soybeans to the cows. Unfortunately, this method only produces organic butter with the same harmful ratio of omega-6 to omega-3 fatty acids and the same mycotoxin risks as conventional butter from grain-fed cows. Mold in our food supply actually prefers organic food, because the food has no chemical fungicides on it. We would choose nonorganic butter from grass-fed cows over organic butter from grain-fed cows anytime, but organic *and* grass-fed are the ultimate for your health. Our family of four eats between one and two sticks of butter every day.

For those who simply won't consider giving up milk, cheese, and yogurt despite the health benefits of doing so, the best choice is to select raw milk and raw-milk cheese and yogurt from grass-fed animals. If raw isn't available or isn't legal in your state, then at least choose grass-fed, and preferably from sheep or goat. Sheep and goat dairy has less allergenic proteins and about 20 percent more butyrate, a type of fat that helps your brain, than cow dairy.

Low-Mercury Fish

In a clean environment, fish is one of the healthiest foods for people to eat. Fish is rich in healthy protein, vitamin D, and omega-3 fatty acids. Due to modern pollution, however, most fish contains levels of mercury and polychlorinated biphenyls (PCBs) that aren't safe. That's why the last chapter recommended avoiding most seafood during pregnancy.

Salmon-Buying Tips

To avoid mercury and other toxins in salmon, it's important to buy wild caught sockeye salmon. Farmed salmon isn't healthy, because it's fed soy and rendered poultry litter and is given high doses of pesticides and antibiotics. Even farmed salmon that contains less mercury than the high-mercury species of salmon is typically higher in contaminants like PCBs, and it is also universally lower in omega-3 compared to wild caught salmon.

Fortunately, there are some types of fish that have a consistently low risk of mercury contamination. Short-lived fish like sardines and anchovies tend to be safe because they don't live long enough for mercury to build up in their bodies. Sardines are a great source of RNA and omega-3 and are very affordable. Although we usually don't eat canned foods, Lana ate about two cans of sardines each week during pregnancy because they're so healthy.

Wild caught sockeye salmon is another safe fish. Its mercury content is extremely low because it lives for a short time, and unlike other types of salmon, it eats only plankton—not other fish, which would expose it to the mercury that those fish absorbed. Many of the plankton that salmon eat are bright red (an indicator of high antioxidant content), which is why sockeye salmon has such a bright, deep orange color compared to other salmon.

Other lower-risk fish are summer flounder, haddock, Petrale sole, tilapia, and wild freshwater sport fish like trout. It's important to check the latest research on mercury contamination in fish published by organizations like the Environmental Working Group, because contamination levels do change over time. Fish that's been tested and verified to be clean of mercury and PCBs is healthy, too, but testing is rare and expensive.

Vegetables and Low-Sugar Fruits

Vegetables are certainly a valuable part of a diet that builds a healthy baby, and we eat lots of them every day. Nonetheless, the reputation vegetables have as health foods should not cause us to overemphasize their importance relative to other Better Baby building blocks.

You may have seen charts showing how many vitamins or minerals are in certain foods and made the conclusion that they should be a major part of your diet. That's reasonable, but clever marketing from food companies like the Whole Foods ANDI score will tell you that foods like kale are superior to eggs and meat.

Since vegetables are often relatively low in calories and high in water and indigestible fiber, this type of chart naturally understates the nutritional value of foods containing healthy fat and protein and overstates the nutritional value of vegetables. That's why, as we noted earlier, this book uses both a food pyramid and a pie chart.

If you buy into this type of food analysis, you'd have to literally eat a bucket full of the top-ranked foods in order to get enough food to support your body and a healthy baby, and you'd still be deficient in healthy fats and proteins.

Almost any green vegetable is going to be healthy for you, but different vegetables have different levels of the various essential minerals and nutrients. The nutrients that are found in most vegetables are folate, dietary fiber, potassium, and magnesium, but vitamin levels vary greatly depending on soil quality and how long ago the vegetable was picked.

We don't eat vegetables just for their nutrients. We also eat them for the protection they offer, because they have powerful preventative effects against cancer and other diseases. But the protective effect is not just for us.

A recent study conducted by the Linus Pauling Institute at Oregon State University found that the mother's intake of cruciferous (the cabbage family) vegetables may provide her baby lifelong protection from cancer. We take this seriously, because cancer is the leading cause of childhood death in the United States today, second only to accidents. This study, one of the first of its kind, suggests that the fight against cancer begins with mother's diet, long before birth. Given what has been discovered about epigenetic effects in the last fifteen years, this makes a lot of sense.

Cruciferous vegetables are a significant part of our diet. They include broccoli, red and green cabbage, brussels sprouts, cauliflower, collard greens, kale, and radishes. Eating these and other fresh vegetables is one of the best ways to consume antioxidants and other compounds that protect both mother and baby from carcinogens. Our other favorite vegetables are asparagus, artichokes, celery, cucumbers, fennel, green beans, dark green lettuce, parsley, spinach, winter squash (like butternut), and summer squash (like zucchini).

All vegetables are not equally healthy, however, because some vegetables are high in sugar and carbohydrates. We recommend eating these infrequently, once a day or less, and having them for dinner not breakfast. Examples of high-sugar vegetables are beets, peas, plantains, potatoes, sweet potatoes and yams, and winter squash. Corn is another "vegetable" (it's really a grain) that's high in carbohydrates. We don't generally recommend corn, except for organic non-GMO corn on the cob as an occasional treat.

You may have noticed that the list of high-sugar vegetables is composed of mostly root vegetables. Carrots are a big exception among root vegetables. High in carotenoids and B vitamins, carrots have a number of well-documented health benefits. In our chapter on supplements, we discuss how the body uses carotenoids to make the perfect amount of vitamin A. The other reason we eat carrots is their ability to help the body eliminate mycotoxins. According to fetal toxicologist Jack Thrasher, "When eaten raw, carrots are efficient colon cleansers, which tone the bowel, reduce the reabsorption of estrogen, and lower cholesterol." You may remember from chapter 4 that many mycotoxins are estrogenic hormone disrupters. Eating raw carrots is a great way to reduce the impact of unwanted estrogens in general, including mycotoxins. We feel a noticeable clarity of mind when we eat them.

Eggplant, peppers (both bell and hot), tomatoes, and potatoes are members of the nightshade family and contain lectins. Lectins are damaging to the lining of your joints and can exacerbate arthritis, and they are also known to cause gut inflammation. With the exception of hot peppers, nightshade vegetables are higher in carbohydrates, so it's better to eat them in smaller quantities. Sensitivity to nightshade vegetables varies from person to person. Lana tried eating them when she was pregnant and quickly learned that she felt better when she avoided eggplant and potatoes but that she felt fine eating peppers and tomatoes. For people who tolerate them well, they can be quite nutritious. For example, hot peppers and tomatoes have valuable nutrients like beta-carotene and lycopene. If you're sensitive, however, removing these from your diet while you're pregnant is a good idea.

Sweet potatoes and yams (there is a slight difference) are not members of the nightshade family, so the warnings about potatoes don't apply to them. However, like other root vegetables, they are high in starch and should not be a large part of your diet because they boost the blood insulin level. As an occasional starchy treat that has a lot of nutrients, try

---

Satisfying Salad Dressing

In our home, no salad is complete without a great dressing that contains healthy fats. We avoid commercial dressings because they are almost universally contaminated with unhealthy oils or chemicals vaguely identified as "spices" or "spice extracts" that usually contain monosodium glutamate.

You can make countless dressings by mixing four basic ingredients:

1. One or more healthy fats
2. Vinegar, lemon juice, or something else acidic
3. An emulsifier—something to help the fat and liquid mix (usually avocado, egg yolk, or non-GMO lecithin)
4. Spices and herbs

Here is our favorite recipe:

½ avocado
2 tablespoons coconut oil
3 tablespoons MCT oil
2 tablespoons apple cider vinegar
1/3 cucumber (medium size)
salt to taste
pinch of xylitol or stevia
fresh cilantro, oregano, or sweet or spicy pepper

Blend to create a thick, creamy dressing that's as full of flavor as it is of nutrients.

---

them with (you guessed it) lots of butter, or with protein, which will help to slow the carbohydrate absorption and reduce the insulin boost.

In general, we advise you to eat your vegetables with substantial amounts of healthy fat and protein. This not only makes the vegetables taste good and feel more filling, it also helps you to absorb more of the nutrients from the vegetables. That's why when we make salad, for example, we use chopped vegetables with a high-nutrient density and add salmon for protein along with avocado, nuts, and a dressing made with MCT oil or olive oil. Without the oils from the high-fat foods and the dressing, the salad simply wouldn't be nutritious enough to provide the vital nutrients a growing fetus needs. It wouldn't satisfy your hunger, either. You'd probably be craving another meal in no time.

Eat Plenty of Vegetables Raw

We advise you to eat a lot of your vegetables—we recommend 75 percent—raw. As the fetus goes through one critical developmental stage after another, there is a constant need for good nutrients, and in most cases these nutrients are more available in raw vegetables than in cooked ones.

Another reason we recommend eating more of your vegetables raw than cooked is that in addition to the fact that raw vegetables keep more of their vitamins and minerals intact, raw vegetables maintain more of their enzymes than do vegetables that are cooked (heated above 116 to 118 degrees Fahrenheit). Enzymes are proteins that make the chemical reactions in your body happen faster and more efficiently. The body uses enzymes not just to digest food but to repair itself.

Some of the enzymes we use we get from vegetables and other foods we eat. But others are manufactured by the pancreas, which makes twenty-two of the body's enzymes. One of the goals of eating raw vegetables is to allow your pancreas to devote more of the energy of its naturally occurring enzymes to keeping your body strong and in good repair, and less to digesting food, so that it can support the healthiest baby.

Many raw-food enthusiasts refer to the enzymes in raw vegetables as "living" enzymes. Enzymes are proteins, so, strictly speaking, they're not live organisms. Nonetheless, they are a strong force in sustaining life.

When we started eating more raw vegetables, we noticed that we felt much more energetic and had better digestion. Our skin improved noticeably. These are good signs of better overall health and are a clear indication that the enzymes are doing their job. Signs of an enzyme deficiency include bloating, belching, gas, bowel disorders, abdominal cramps, heartburn, and food allergies. If you experience any of these symptoms on a regular basis, eating more raw vegetables can help to alleviate them, provided you're not allergic to any of the vegetables and not suffering from a systemic yeast infection.

A German study concluded that "uncooked food is an integral component of human nutrition, and is a necessary precondition for an intact immune system." The study found that raw food has antibiotic, antiallergenic, anti-inflammatory, tumor-protective, and other positive, immune-strengthening effects on the body. It also concluded that raw food should be viewed as a "useful adjunct to drugs in the treatment of allergic, rheumatic, and infectious diseases." We would add that an intact immune system is particularly important for fertility, pregnancy, and the prevention of autism-related immune overreaction in babies.

Nevertheless, you will find that some recognized authorities (including many doctors) recommend that pregnant women avoid eating raw vegetables entirely because of the risk of bacteria (such as *Salmonella*) or parasites (usually parasite eggs). These can be harmful for the mother and the baby, and it's true that cooking kills most of them. Fortunately, you don't have to sacrifice the advantages of eating a lot of your vegetables raw, because there's an easy way to kill any bacteria and parasite eggs on the outside of vegetables without cooking them: you simply add about ten drops of Lugol's iodine or GSE (as we explained earlier with raw eggs) to about a quart of water and mix, and soak your raw vegetables in the solution for a minute or two. This will sterilize the vegetables without affecting their taste or destroying any enzymes or nutrients.

You can rinse the vegetables afterward or enjoy the health benefits of added iodine or GSE. If raw vegetables are washed properly, the benefits of eating them during pregnancy are far greater than the questionable benefits of avoiding them. There is no need to spend money on chemical vegetable-wash sprays from the store. Most won't disinfect as well as simple iodine.

Eat Some Vegetables Cooked

As we noted earlier, we try to eat at least 75 percent of our vegetables raw, but lightly cooking some vegetables can make their nutrients easier to digest. For example, the beta-carotene in broccoli, carrots, and spinach is more easily absorbed into the body if they've been steamed. Spinach and rhubarb are healthier when cooked, because cooking deactivates the unhealthy oxalic acid they contain. It's also easier for the body to get lycopene from tomatoes that have been cooked lightly.

When you do cook vegetables, baking, broiling, steaming, and boiling are better techniques than frying and grilling, because the risk for oxidation is much lower. We don't sauté vegetables in oil, because heated oils oxidize easily. When the vegetables are done cooking, we add either butter from grass-fed cows or a healthy oil like olive or coconut; this way, the oil won't oxidize.

The following plants should never be eaten raw, because they are toxic unless cooked: buckwheat greens, cassava (including cassava flour), legumes, and parsnips. Naming and discussing the toxins in each of these is beyond the scope of this book, but the evidence is clear that pregnant women should avoid them.

Digestive Enzyme Supplements

Taking a high-quality digestive enzyme supplement can help your body digest cooked foods. Raw foods have their naturally occurring enzymes intact, so there is no need to take supplemental enzymes if you are having only salad, for instance. Digestive enzyme supplements don't replace every enzyme found in raw foods, but they reduce the burden on your body when you eat cooked food. There are a dizzying array of digestive enzymes on the market, some much more useful than others. We recommend the higher-quality ones on www.betterbabybook.com.

Avocado Power

Avocados have a long history as a food—they were originally cultivated by the Mayans and the Aztecs. Avocados are rich in vitamins E and K, potassium, folate, and monounsaturated fats, which are essential for heart health and low cholesterol. Vitamin K is a central component in blood coagulation, and it has been linked to increased bone mass. In fact, a form of vitamin K2 is a recognized treatment for osteoporosis in Japan. Vitamin K may also play a role in preventing Alzheimer's disease as well as liver and prostate cancer.

As a good source of potassium, avocados help to regulate blood pressure and prevent circulatory complications. Both potassium and the folate in avocados have been linked with a reduced rate of stroke.

There is particular value in putting avocado in your salad. The *Journal of Nutrition* published a study confirming that the carotenoids in salad vegetables like lettuce and carrots are more bioavailable when consumed with the monounsaturated fats contained in avocados. The participants in this study absorbed far more carotenoids from a salad of spinach, lettuce, and carrots when it was accompanied by even small amounts of avocado. So eating avocado with your salad makes the rest of the salad a lot healthier for you—and your baby!

We rely on avocados for a significant portion of our healthy monounsaturated fat because they are convenient, because guacamole is easy to find at restaurants, and because half an avocado blended into almost anything will give it a pleasant, creamy texture. Our family of four goes through about fifteen to twenty avocados every week, about one per person per day!

About Juicing

If you have a hard time eating enough vegetables, consider drinking fresh vegetable juice. The juice will contain most of the enzymes, minerals, and vitamins present in the vegetables. Some juicing methods do a better job than others of preserving enzymes, but all vegetable juice will be beneficial as long as it is not pasteurized. Vegetable juice does, however, lack much of the dietary fiber that vegetables themselves contain. So if you do choose to get most of your raw vegetables through juice, and if you have a problem with bowel regularity (common in pregnancy), taking a dietary fiber supplement like pectin may be a good idea.

We aren't against juicing. Although it's not as healthy as eating whole vegetables, if that's the only way you can consume raw vegetables, by all means do it. But we advise that you work with a nutritionist or, at minimum, buy a good book on vegetable juicing, because there are lots of things you need to know about the pros and cons of juicing and how to get the most from it.

Low-Sugar Fruits

The lowest-sugar fruits are lemons and limes, followed by blackberries, cranberries, grapefruit, passion fruit, raspberries, and strawberries. When you are going to eat fruit, these are the best choices.

Fruits with an average amount of sugar are apples, apricots, blueberries, cantaloupe, cherries, kiwi, nectarines, oranges, papaya, peaches, pears, pineapple, and plums. It's best to eat these fruits infrequently, as a treat once or twice a week.

Fruits that are very high in sugar really don't belong in a healthy diet for pregnant women. These are bananas, dates, figs, grapes, guava, lychee, mangoes, melons, persimmon, pomegranate, tangerines, raisins, and any other dried fruits. If you do eat these fruits, use them in very small amounts to enhance the flavor of other healthier foods.

Keep in mind that fruit sugar primarily comes in the form of fructose, the sugar that's most damaging to our health. This is why fruits and vegetables are in separate categories on the Better Baby food pyramid.

Nourishing Nuts

Nuts are among the most dense, nutrient-packed foods that nature offers. They are especially valuable for their healthy fatty acids, proteins, and trace minerals. In this section, we'll discuss how to buy, handle, store, and prepare nuts.

The nuts we recommend eating are almonds, cashews, chestnuts, hazelnuts, macadamia nuts, pecans, pine nuts, and walnuts.

Of course, it goes without saying that if you're allergic to nuts, you should avoid them, especially when you're pregnant.

"Nuts" That Aren't Nuts

You may notice that soy "nuts," peanuts, and corn "nuts" are not on the list. These are not really nuts at all—they're legumes (soybeans, peanuts) or a grain (corn). Our reasons for avoiding soy, peanuts, and corn are detailed in chapter 4.

The nutritional benefits of nuts come with some level of risk. Nuts are particularly susceptible to infection with toxic molds, which produce mycotoxins. For that reason, it's ideal to buy whole, raw, shelled nuts that have always been refrigerated or frozen—if you can find them.

Nuts should be raw, because roasting them will chemically alter their nutritive value and fat composition and reduce their positive health effects. Also, nuts contain the amino acid asparagine, which when roasted produces acrylamide, known to cause cancer in animals and believed to be a carcinogen for humans as well.

Nuts should be refrigerated because they are high in fat and become rancid when exposure to warm air causes the fats to oxidize. Storing nuts in the refrigerator or the freezer prevents this from happening. It also protects them from their susceptibility to mold.

Try to find a health-food store that sells whole, organic, raw, refrigerated nuts. Only the best health-food stores carry them, however, and they are expensive. So if you can't find a store that carries them or can't afford to pay for them, we recommend that at a minimum you should buy nuts that are whole and not chopped, because the outer layer of the kernel can protect the nut from mold. It's even better to buy nuts in the shell, because the shell protects the nut.

There's a lot of overlap among the different kinds of nuts and their nutritional values. For example, almost all nuts are rich in monounsaturated fats, which are healthy for your circulatory system and have been shown to reduce the risk of cardiovascular disease. But each nut also offers its own particular health benefits. Here are the specific benefits of each nut (the nuts are listed in alphabetical order):

- *Almonds* are an excellent source of copper, vitamin E, magnesium, manganese, phosphorus, riboflavin (vitamin B2), and tryptophan. This unique vitamin and mineral profile helps to reduce stress and control after-meal blood sugar surges. Keeping blood sugar under control supports a stable energy level throughout the day. Almonds are also high in monounsaturated fats that reduce the risk of heart disease and promote a healthy cholesterol level. They're also relatively resistant to molds and rarely contain mycotoxins. Raw almond butter is a great way to include almonds in your daily menu.

- *Brazil nuts* are rich in selenium, a mineral that is central to proper thyroid function, but are very heavily contaminated with mycotoxins. We avoid them for that reason.

- *Cashews* contain high amounts of copper and magnesium. Copper deficiency has been linked to several health problems like anemia and white blood cell disorders.

- *Chestnuts* are lower in fat than other nuts and are higher in starches and sugars. They are a great source of essential minerals, including iron, zinc, copper, and manganese. We do not eat chestnuts often, however, because of their carbohydrate content.

- *Hazelnuts* are one of the richest sources of vitamin E in all of nature. The vitamin E in hazelnuts is more biologically active and useful to your body than synthetic vitamin E supplements. There are eight different forms of vitamin E, and hazelnuts contain most of them.

- *Macadamia nuts* are one of the best sources of monounsaturated fats. An astounding 80 percent of the fat in macadamia nuts is monounsaturated (that's even higher than olive oil), and much of it is omega-7 fatty acids, which are known for maintaining skin health. Studies have proved that macadamia nuts lower LDL (bad) cholesterol.

- *Pecans* are loaded with great fats, vitamins, and nutrients, especially thiamine, zinc, and manganese. They also contain more antioxidants by volume than any other nut.

- *Pine nuts* are a great source of memory-boosting omega-9 fatty acids, iron, and magnesium.

- *Pistachios* have a nutrition profile that rivals all the nuts we've discussed so far. They're richest in copper, manganese, and phosphorus. Pistachios also contain lots of folate, biotin, thiamine, niacin, riboflavin, and pantothenic acid—all of which are part of the vitamin B family. Pistachios are the only nuts that contain significant amounts of carotenoids, lutein, and zeaxanthin. They're also higher in dietary fiber than most other nuts. Pistachios do tend to have a higher risk of mold, so inspect them before eating them.

- *Walnuts* are the unqualified kings of omega-3 fatty acid content, and they have substantial omega-6 as well. Like the other nuts, walnuts have a lot of vitamins and minerals. If you choose to eat only one of the nuts on this list, choose walnuts, but don't cook with them because that will oxidize their oils and create free radicals.

Collagen Keeps It All Together

Collagen is the central building block for a variety of structurally important tissues, including bone, cartilage, tendons, and ligaments. Collagen is also found in skin, other organs, and even blood. It is the most abundant fibrous protein in the human body.

Even though our bodies are designed to manufacture collagen, they need the right combination of amino acids, vitamins, and minerals to do so. Since our bodies will selectively use these materials to meet short-term needs for other processes, a shortage may develop, and poorly formed collagen will result. Our program calls for a pregnant woman to add plenty of high-quality collagen to her diet, along with collagen building blocks like vitamin C. We feel confident that since Lana took plenty of collagen throughout both pregnancies, our children's bones and organs had plenty of body-building collagen available in utero. We also believe that collagen supplementation, along with a high healthy-fat diet, is what prevented Lana from getting even a single stretch mark despite having two children after age forty.

When most people think of collagen, they think of soft skin, shiny hair, and full lips. They are absolutely right—collagen helps you to have all of those assets. Collagen is a key component of hair, skin, and nails.

As hormones fluctuate during the course of pregnancy, a woman's skin and hair change dramatically. Taking extra collagen keeps them beautiful.

But a little-known and very important fact about collagen is its function as a semiconductor of electricity. Why is that a good thing?

Collagen's ability to conduct electricity inside the body makes it central to the communication between cells, which leads to optimum growth and healing. This may sound a little far-out, but it's not. The research that discovered this led to a new way to heal bone fractures in limbs that would have previously required amputation, and it therefore also led to two Nobel Prize nominations.

Healthy joints that are full of properly hydrated collagen serve to facilitate the electrical flow required for good cell communication. Perhaps the most important everyday function of this intercellular communication is that it helps the cells work together to eliminate their own toxic waste products. The most noticeable health effects of the efficient disposal of toxins will be smoother skin, properly functioning joints, and higher energy—exactly the effects that we noticed from taking two or three tablespoons of a nearly flavorless collagen supplement in a smoothie every day. We give our children supplemental collagen, too, which we started doing as soon as they were able to drink anything other than breast milk.

The average American diet usually doesn't provide enough of the amino acids required to make optimal levels of well-formed collagen. Just as a carpenter can't make tables without wood, the body can't make collagen without the necessary raw materials. When the body can't make enough collagen, it becomes more susceptible to injury and heals more slowly. Even if you drink enough water, your body has a hard time staying hydrated when there is a shortage of collagen in your tissues. This can lead to a buildup of toxins and related problems, especially when you must meet the new demands of pregnancy. Pregnant mothers will therefore be particularly vulnerable to the effects of collagen deficiency. Evidence of collagen deficiency can be seen in stretch marks, easy bruising, brittle hair that falls out after delivery, sagging skin, and even nosebleeds.

There are dozens of forms of collagen supplementation on the market, including common gelatin. The collagen we believe to be the best for you is called hydrolyzed collagen, or collagen hydrolysate, because it is the form most easily absorbed by the body.

But please note that we are recommending it as a supplement to and not a replacement for other kinds of protein. In the 1970s, hydrolyzed collagen became a very popular dietary supplement. Unfortunately, many companies promoted it as part of an extremely low-calorie liquid protein diet aimed at weight loss, and they misrepresented it as being a legitimate "sole" source of protein. Nothing could be further from the truth. Although hydrolyzed collagen contains the amino acids that many people need (and are deficient in), it's an incomplete protein and does not contain a number of essential amino acids. So hydrolyzed collagen should never be considered a complete protein for anyone, least of all for a pregnant woman. But it is an excellent supplement to build healthy tissues.

The source of collagen and its processing method is very important. Most companies get their collagen from factory-farmed animals, which provide collagen that is of lower quality. Or they subject the collagen to intensive heating or acid washing, which destroys many of the building blocks for a baby's joints, eyes, and heart. That is not good news! We maintain a list of high-quality, safe hydrolyzed collagen brands at www .betterbabybook.com/collagen and suggest that you consult the list before buying supplemental collagen.

Since much of the protein in the human body is made of collagen, a mother's body will naturally need a lot of it to construct her baby's body properly. Here is what you can expect from adding collagen to your diet.

The structural materials and nutrients in hydrolyzed collagen go directly to making stronger cartilage, ligaments, tendons, bones, and disks. This means a more resilient, flexible body that is less prone to injury and that heals faster when it *is* injured. It also means giving your baby the ideal building blocks for growing in the womb. It means better bone growth for your baby and denser bones for you as an adult.

Individuals who are prone to repetitive joint injury, pain, and discomfort will see a marked decrease in joint inflammation and pain and will feel much better, because musculoskeletal injuries heal faster and the body becomes stronger.

After a person reaches age twenty-five, collagen production declines at a rate of 1 to 1.5 percent per year. As the collagen level falls, the connective tissues begin to deteriorate. Taking hydrolyzed collagen is especially helpful for older expecting mothers, because it helps them to stay fit during the process of building a baby.

Hydrolyzed collagen's high glycine content also assists the liver in handling toxins and keeping them away from your baby.

The mental benefits of collagen supplementation include greater alertness, better concentration, balanced mood, improved energy, and an increased sense of well-being. This helps control a mother's stress. When the mom is happy, the baby is happy!

The Only Good Soy Is Soy Lecithin

As you know, we do not regard soy or soy products as healthy foods, but soy lecithin is the exception to this rule. Luckily for pregnant women, lecithin thickens soybean oil too much, so soy manufacturers pull the lecithin out of the oil and sell it as a dietary supplement. Lecithin is just another name for "sticky fats." You'll find different forms of it in eggs, meat, and (in small amounts) many other foods.

Supplementing with lecithin during pregnancy is valuable for you and your baby, because lecithin is high in choline: 13 percent of lecithin is pure choline. As we explained in our discussion of eggs, choline is critical to a child's brain development. In one group of studies, the choline in lecithin reduced the level of homocysteine, an amino acid that in excess has been associated with neural tube defects. Supplementing with lecithin (choline) is a great way to keep your homocysteine level under control.

Pregnant women should get at least 450 milligrams of choline per day and nursing mothers at least 550 milligrams per day. We recommend taking two tablespoons of granular lecithin daily, because that will provide about 500 milligrams of choline (eating eggs will also help you and your baby get the choline you need). Note that any soy lecithin you buy should be labeled as certified organic, or at least non-GMO, because soy is usually genetically modified. As of 2010, we could find only one manufacturer of organic soy lecithin in the United States.

Soy lecithin comes in small granules and has a mild nutty flavor. It should not be cooked, because the omega-6 will oxidize easily; you should also store it in the refrigerator. Lecithin has the amazing ability to transform just about any smoothie, salad dressing, or homemade coconut-based "ice cream" into a thick, creamy delight.

For those of you who are allergic to soy, unless you have an extreme anaphylactic reaction, you aren't likely to be allergic to soy lecithin. Most of the allergen proteins contained in soy are removed during the manufacturing process, making allergic reactions rare. Nonetheless, if you're allergic to soy, it's important to monitor yourself for allergic reactions when you first try soy lecithin. Sunflower lecithin is even better.

Cilantro

Cilantro has many health benefits, including strong antibacterial effects against *Salmonella*. A study published in the *Journal of Agriculture and Food Chemistry* found that cilantro was twice as effective at killing *Salmonella* as Gentamicin, the commercial drug that is commonly used to fight *Salmonella* infection. Cilantro is a natural chelator, which means that it may protect you and your baby from heavy metals like mercury and lead. This is particularly useful when you eat fish that might have mercury in it.

Cilantro also functions as a digestive agent, prevents nausea (good for dealing with morning sickness), is an anti-inflammatory, relieves intestinal gas, helps to control blood sugar, and optimizes the cholesterol level. Cilantro is a great source of dietary fiber, iron, manganese, and magnesium. Putting cilantro on salad or in guacamole or cooking with it is a great way to incorporate this powerful herb into your diet. Fresh organic cilantro is ideal.

Ginger

Ginger has been used medicinally and as a food for thousands of years, and research is bearing out its efficacy. In 2009, the *Journal of Alternative and Complementary Medicine* published a study showing that ginger decreases nausea and vomiting during pregnancy. Sixty-seven pregnant women with nausea and vomiting symptoms each received either 250 milligrams of ginger or a placebo for four days. The participants who took ginger showed a marked improvement over those who received the placebo.

Eating ginger is a good way to aid the digestion of fats and proteins and to reduce gas. Ginger neutralizes the acids in the digestive system that cause nausea, cramps, vomiting, and diarrhea. Ginger also reduces inflammation, stimulates circulation, and acts as a natural antihistamine and antifungal.

Ginger's health benefits come from its oils, gingerol and shogaol. These oils give ginger its distinctive taste.

We sometimes grate ginger root into our salad dressing or use it to make Thai-style sauces, which call for coconut milk, too. We also make fresh ginger tea. To brew your own, buy a large ginger root (preferably organic) at your local grocery store. Peel the skin off with a vegetable peeler and cut the root into thin strips. Heat a quart or so of water in a saucepan until it comes to a rolling boil, add the ginger strips, reduce the heat, and let the ginger simmer for about twenty minutes. Adding a dash of fresh lemon juice at the end is a nice touch. Of course, you can just use ginger tea bags, but making your own tea is easy, fun, and delicious.

White Rice

If you're going to eat any grain, we recommend rice, because even though it isn't immune to molds, it's resistant and therefore less likely to be contaminated with mycotoxins than grains like corn and wheat. Organically grown white rice is about as healthy as a pure carbohydrate can get. We find that Japanese mochi made from pounded sweet rice is an amazing baked treat for Sunday mornings, when we consciously choose to "cheat" and eat carbs.

Whey Protein

Whey protein is a white powder supplement that contains a diverse blend of essential and nonessential amino acids. These amino acids give your body the building blocks it needs both to maintain itself and to grow a healthy baby. During pregnancy, your body demands a constant supply of protein to give your baby a good foundation, and supplementing with whey protein helps ensure that all of your protein bases are covered, since not every meal will deliver the protein you need. High-quality whey proteins also normalize weight, helping overweight people to lose weight and underweight people to gain it.

There are a number of things to watch out for when buying whey protein, because there's a lot of unhealthy, poor-quality protein products out there. Many are geared toward body builders and contain extra sugar, flavoring, and harmful chemicals. Many are processed in such a way that they cause the proteins to become unusable inside the body, or even harmful. Whey protein concentrates are a bad idea. They often contain casein and lactose, which we have already discussed under the topic of milk.

During pregnancy, you should look for whey protein isolate that is labeled "low-temperature processed" and "nonhydrolyzed." Low-temperature processing preserves the natural forms of the proteins and prevents them from being damaged (denatured) from high heat. The natural forms are healthier for the body. For this reason, we never cook with whey protein or mix it into very hot liquid. Whey protein from grass-fed cows is ideal, but it's expensive. If you have allergies, goat whey protein may be better for you than the standard bovine product.

You can find a list of whey protein brands that meet our standards at our website, www.betterbabybook.com/whey.

Morning Smoothie with Whey Protein

This recipe makes a smoothie that is on par with the finest ice cream milk shakes. Our kids love this, and our guests routinely rave about our smoothies.

    1 tablespoon or more xylitol or stevia to taste
    1 tablespoon MCT oil
    1 tablespoon organic coconut oil or ¼ can coconut cream
    1–2 raw egg yolks (discard the whites)
    1–2 tablespoons non-GMO soy lecithin
    ice

1–6 tablespoons water, depending on how thick you like your smoothies
To add flavor, use one or more of the following:

1 lime, peeled

berries of your choice, frozen or fresh

vanilla extract

cinnamon (helps to control blood sugar level)

raw organic cocoa powder

2 tablespoons whey protein

2 tablespoons collagen protein (optional)

Blend all ingredients except the whey and collagen proteins until smooth. Then add the two proteins and blend just until smooth, being careful not to overblend the second time. Overblending can damage some of the delicate whey protein structures. This will make the smoothie less beneficial for you, though not harmful.

If you're in a rush and just need to get some protein into your body for quick energy because you don't have time to eat a real meal, put 1 to 3 tablespoons of whey protein in a few ounces of water, add 1 to 2 tablespoons of MCT oil, shake, and drink.

Xylitol and Stevia

Xylitol is a type of sweetener found naturally in the fiber of a variety of fruits and vegetables. Since xylitol does not raise the blood sugar level and contains no fructose, it's our sweetener of choice. It also contributes to dental health and has been shown to be an effective treatment for osteoporosis. It's completely safe to use while you're pregnant, and it can even prevent the transfer of harmful bacteria from a mother to her baby.

Eating too much xylitol before your body gets used to making the enzymes you need to digest it can lead to bloating or diarrhea, so start on xylitol slowly and then build up, backing off if you get unpleasant symptoms. If xylitol doesn't work out so well for you the first time, don't get discouraged—your body will definitely adapt to it over time. And once you've adapted, you'll get all the benefits of a healthy, satisfying sweet-ener that replaces sugar very well in most recipes. Xylitol from hard-wood, not corn, is best.

Stevia is another healthy sweetener that's low in carbohydrates and doesn't raise the blood sugar level. We prefer xylitol, because stevia tastes bitter to us, just as it does for many people. But some people love the taste of stevia, and from a health perspective, it's a great choice.

Dark Chocolate and Cocoa Butter

In recent years, chocolate has become known for its health benefits. Chocolate is high in antioxidants like flavonoids and catechins. Flavo-noids optimize blood pressure and increase blood flow by helping the body to create nitric oxide—probably one reason that chocolate has a reputation for being an aphrodisiac! Chocolate also contains serotonin and stimulates the production of endorphins, both of which improve mood and make you feel better.

Chocolate is a source of some healthy fats. An August 2010 study confirmed that chocolate optimizes cholesterol levels without detri-mental side effects. The study participants ate forty-five grams of 85 percent cacao chocolate every day for eight weeks. That's about half of a bar each day, quite a bit of chocolate! But note that what they were eating was nearly pure chocolate, very low in sugar, and free of milk.

Chocolate does contain caffeine, but not much. One ounce of dark chocolate has about 20 milligrams of caffeine. There are 60 to 120 milligrams of caffeine in a cup of brewed coffee and 45 milligrams in a cup of black tea. We know that it's important to limit caffeine intake during pregnancy, but if chocolate is consumed moderately, the small amount of caffeine it contains will not be enough to make a difference for most people. Lana ate a few squares of very dark chocolate two or three times per week while pregnant. We think that chocolate's healthy fat content and its ability to reduce Lana's stress benefited our children. We know it benefited Lana!

Tips for Buying and Storing Chocolate

When we say chocolate, we do mean chocolate—not the milk and sugar that are often added to chocolate in such large amounts. Unfortunately, milk chocolate, truffles, chocolate confections, chocolate candies, and the like usually contain way too much sugar.

To get the chocolate and avoid the milk and sugar, we recommend only 80 percent or higher dark chocolate. Dark chocolate with almonds or other healthy nuts is one of our favorites. We particularly enjoy eating Swiss or other European chocolates, which are produced at a higher standard than most domestic brands.

We also eat pure raw organic cocoa butter, which is just the healthy fat from chocolate. Cocoa butter shavings in hot drinks make a nice mocha flavor.

Chocolate stays fresh if you store it in the refrigerator or the freezer after you open it.

The Better Baby Book Nutrition Guidelines

We have just presented you with an almost dizzying array of information, some of which challenges conventional dietary wisdom. Please don't feel like you need to do everything in this chapter to give your baby a good start in life. The reason our book is called *The Better Baby Book* instead of *The Perfect Baby Book* is that your goal should be improvement rather than perfection. The pursuit of perfection can only lead to feelings of failure, which will undermine rather than enhance your health.

That said, the information in this chapter can help you to be more conscious of your diet's effect on both your own body and your baby's growing body. Although our diet is designed for a healthy pregnancy, it is equally suited to helping your body create optimal breast milk and to giving you the energy and stamina you need to wake up several times a night to nourish your little one with that breast milk.

We've included the diagrams to help you track our recommendations and decide which are right for you. So you can see how healthy foods compare to unhealthy ones, we include the good foods from this chapter as well as the foods to avoid mentioned in chapter 4. We also explain how costly or difficult it is to buy, prepare, and eat foods the Better Baby way, and we give hints to make things easier for you.

Proteins

Meat from grass-fed animals costs a lot at restaurants or from gourmet butchers, but if you order it online, it costs little more than beef from grain-fed cows from the average butcher. For one adult, high-end protein powders cost about a dollar per day.

If you cook at home or pack your own lunch, there's no difference in convenience. If you eat out, it may be harder (as well as more expensive) to find meat from grass-fed animals or the recommended kinds of seafood.

Protein Hints

- Eat eggs poached or soft-boiled with runny yolks to preserve choline and omega-3 for your baby's nervous system. Farmers' market or free-range organic eggs are best.

- Eating meat from grass-fed animals once a day will do wonders for your health. As easy to prepare as other meats, it's available

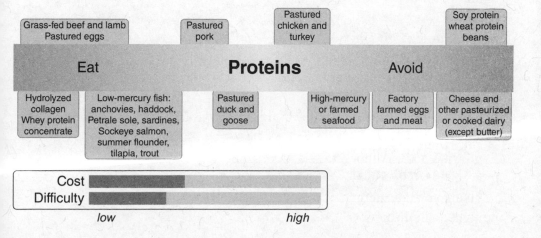

at many farmers' markets, from lots of good butchers, at most Whole Foods stores, or online in bulk.

- We take two to four tablespoons of hydrolyzed collagen every day, in a smoothie or just in water. It has very high health benefits but is somewhat costly compared to whey, which we also take sometimes.

- One or two tablespoons of whey protein concentrate added to a smoothie or water is a fast, easy source of protein, but it's not necessary if you are eating meat and eggs and taking collagen.

Oils and Fats

It does cost more to "live off the fat of the land," but it's one of the most important recommendations in this book. High-end fat sources are expensive because they are highly sought. Choosing your fats wisely will change your life and improve your baby's future.

Using the right healthy fats at home is easy, but many chain restaurants don't even serve pure butter anymore, instead favoring a mix of margarine and butter. Restaurants usually use unhealthy oils (like canola) for cooking, too. Since eating healthy oils and fats usually means cooking at home, this can be difficult.

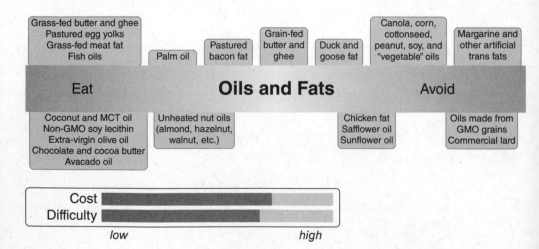

Oil and Fat Hints

- Olive oil is great in salad dressing. We drizzle it over cooked vegetables sometimes, too, but we never cook with it because cooking spoils the oil's health benefits.

- Cooking with butter from grass-fed cows minimizes oxidation and tastes good, too! To minimize oxidation you can also cook with expeller-pressed coconut oil or with MCT oil, which are both flavorless.

- Blend coconut oil or MCT oil into salad dressings and sauces to get the key healthy fats they contain. Coconut milk, a source of healthy coconut oil, goes great in smoothies and Asian soups. Fresh young coconuts are also a delectable way to get the health benefits of coconut.

- Adding a spoonful of non-GMO soy lecithin to any drink, smoothie, or salad dressing gives your baby brain-building choline.

Vegetables and Fruits

Some of the healthiest vegetables, like cabbage, cauliflower, collard greens, and kale, are also some of the cheapest vegetables. It takes some work to buy, wash, and prepare fresh vegetables, but it's definitely worth the effort.

Vegetable and Fruit Hints

- Avocados are a key source of Better Baby building blocks, they satisfy your appetite, and they're very fast to cut up and eat. They're also cheap if you buy them in bulk. Overall, they're one of our absolute favorites.

- If you're craving something sweet, low-sugar fruits like raspberries are a great choice. But remember, eating sugar makes you crave more sugar and won't give you long-lasting energy the way that healthy fat will.

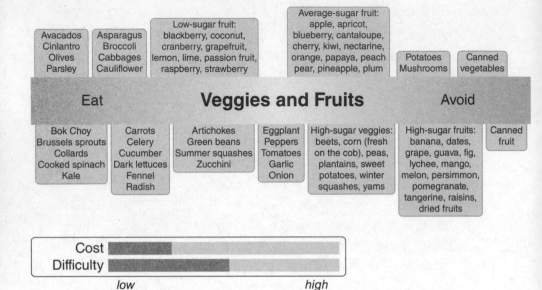

Eat	Veggies and Fruits					Avoid

Eat:
- Avacados, Cinlantro, Olives, Parsley
- Asparagus, Broccoli, Cabbages, Cauliflower
- Low-sugar fruit: blackberry, coconut, cranberry, grapefruit, lemon, lime, passion fruit, raspberry, strawberry
- Average-sugar fruit: apple, apricot, blueberry, cantaloupe, cherry, kiwi, nectarine, orange, papaya, peach, pear, pineapple, plum

Avoid:
- Potatoes, Mushrooms
- Canned vegetables

Eat:
- Bok Choy, Brussels sprouts, Collards, Cooked spinach, Kale
- Carrots, Celery, Cucumber, Dark lettuces, Fennel, Radish
- Artichokes, Green beans, Summer squashes, Zucchini
- Eggplant, Peppers, Tomatoes, Garlic, Onion
- High-sugar veggies: beets, corn (fresh on the cob), peas, plantains, sweet potatoes, winter squashes, yams

Avoid:
- High-sugar fruits: banana, dates, grape, guava, fig, lychee, mango, melon, persimmon, pomegranate, tangerine, raisins, dried fruits
- Canned fruit

Cost (low to high)
Difficulty (low to high)

- Making salads and salad dressings is easier with a blender or a food processor.
- If you have difficulty eating lots of vegetables, try chopping or grating them into coleslaw-like mixtures or juicing them.

Nuts and Legumes

As a quick snack, nuts are more expensive than pretzels, chips, and other unhealthy alternatives, but the health benefits make them an excellent

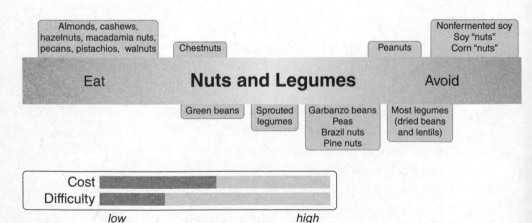

Eat	Nuts and Legumes				Avoid

Eat:
- Almonds, cashews, hazelnuts, macadamia nuts, pecans, pistachios, walnuts
- Chestnuts

Avoid:
- Peanuts
- Nonfermented soy, Soy "nuts", Corn "nuts"

- Green beans
- Sprouted legumes
- Garbanzo beans, Peas, Brazil nuts, Pine nuts
- Most legumes (dried beans and lentils)

Cost (low to high)
Difficulty (low to high)

choice. Adding nuts to your diet is simple—they're easy to carry around with you for snacking on the go, no preparation is required, and they're widely available.

Nut and Legume Hints

- Almond butter spread on celery is a great snack and a fast, easy source of healthy fats and energy.

- It's true that beans and lentils contain healthy protein. Unfortunately, however, they're full of lectins that cause health problems for lots of people. That's why we avoided them during pregnancy. If you'd like to enjoy beans, there are supplements on the market that deactivate lectins and make beans a bit healthier. We maintain a list of quality lectin-blocking supplements on our website, www.betterbabybook.com/lectins.

- Lots of soy products are marketed as health foods. Don't be deceived—they're terrible for you!

Grains

Most grains are cheap, but it's better to avoid them, whether they're refined or whole. The difficulty with grains isn't in preparing them or finding the right ones. The difficulty is in avoiding them. It's hard to avoid grains, because they're so common in the American diet, and it takes a conscious effort to stop eating them. But if you stick to it for thirty days, you'll find a whole new level of wellness.

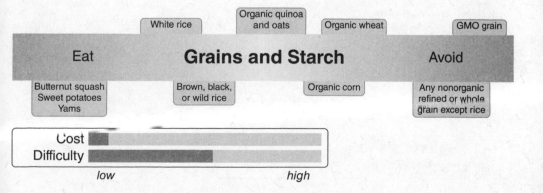

Grain Hints

- White rice is the healthiest option you have for grains. Even this option is high in carbohydrates, though.

- Pressure-cooking grains is smart, because the pressure destroys a number of mold toxins.

- We rarely eat grains, because avoiding them makes us feel much better.

Dairy

Butter from grass-fed cows is marginally more expensive than organic butter, but European brands are sometimes cheaper. Expensive or not, the best, healthiest butter still adds up to only a fraction of your overall food costs and is well worth it. Finding butter from grass-fed cows at grocery stores is usually easy, but it's not available at most restaurants, where your best bet is regular butter or olive oil.

Dairy Hints

- Adding plenty of butter to almost anything makes it delicious— including soups, sauces, and gravies.

- Butter from Ireland and New Zealand is naturally from grass-fed cows even when it's not organic. Using butter from these countries is a great way to get your butter at a lower cost.

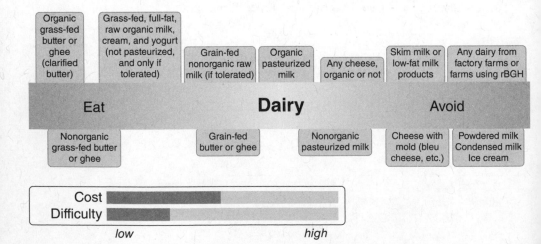

- Avoid cheese—its protein is particularly hard on the body, and it stores mycotoxins.
- It's better to skip dairy in a meal rather than eat it from questionable sources.

Spices and Flavorings

It costs very little to buy the dried herbs listed in the diagram (or to grow your own fresh herbs), and it adds a lot to the taste of your food. Switching to healthy spices is simple when cooking at home, but it's very difficult to know what spices you're getting when you eat at restaurants.

Spice and Flavoring Hints

- Ginger tea is a great way to stave off morning sickness and improve digestion.
- Cilantro is inexpensive and does a great job of helping digestion and binding toxins like mercury. We usually give cilantro a quick wash, chop, and add a little into our salads.

Sweeteners and Sugars

Healthy sugars cost more than white granulated sugar, but the benefits are massive. Using them at home is not hard to do, and there is plenty of recipe help available online.

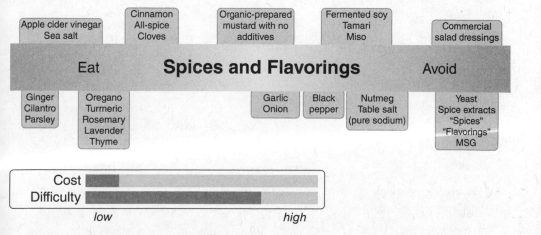

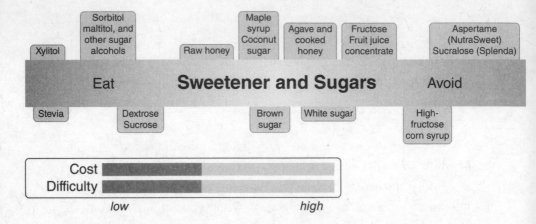

Since most processed and restaurant food has corn syrup or granulated sugar, avoiding these is less convenient but very achievable without a lot of effort. Choosing food wisely is a habit but not a chore.

Sweetener and Sugar Hints

- Watch out for hidden sugars in salad dressing, tomato sauce, and other canned or bottled foods.
- Xylitol works anywhere sugar would work, except it won't caramelize.
- If you're new to xylitol, use it sparingly at first and give your body a week or two to get used to making the enzymes you need to digest it.
- Many sweeteners like agave are promoted as healthy because they raise insulin less. However, they contain large amounts of fructose, the most damaging sugar. Agave has more fructose than corn syrup does.
- We exclusively use xylitol or stevia at home and keep a little raw honey for special occasions.
- Xylitol should come from American hardwood, not from corn.

Cooking

Learning to cook at lower temperatures is not hard to do, but for many people it represents a change in habit, and, of course, cooking more slowly takes longer.

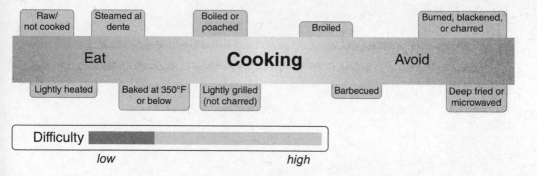

Cooking Hints

- If the food looks blackened or browned, you've damaged the proteins and nutrients, which can cause inflammation.

- Grilling can be acceptable if the food is far enough from the coals or gas to cook gently.

- Remember that meat from grass-fed animals takes about one-third less time to cook than meat from conventional factory-farmed animals.

6

Fertility

The same recommendations we make throughout this book for a healthy pregnancy also boost fertility. Detoxing, eating the right diet, taking the right supplements, and reducing stress boost fertility and make a healthy baby; so do drinking clean water and breathing clean air; making sure you're free of disease; avoiding caffeine, tobacco, and alcohol and simply wanting to have a baby. So in our program, addressing fertility isn't much different from preparing for pregnancy and being pregnant.

Our diet boosts fertility because it's low in sugar and high in healthy fats. The low-sugar intake is important for fertility, because high sugar intake keeps your insulin level high, which disrupts your hormone levels and interferes with fertility in a number of ways. Chromium, magnesium, and N-acetyl-cysteine (NAC) supplementation can help the body to recover from high sugar intake. Eating plenty of healthy fats is important, because women need plenty of energy to sustain a pregnancy. Without it, conception can be difficult, and sometimes ovulation stops.

At the same time, obesity can contribute to infertility. Unhealthy synthetic trans fats can cause ovulatory infertility even if eaten very sparingly (as low as 2 percent of one's total caloric intake). That's just one medium-size order of french fries from your local fast-food restaurant. Also, keep an eye on foods that promote inflammation, like grains, dairy, and oils high in omega-6. Inflammation can create an environment in the body that makes conception difficult.

There are a few key fertility supplements besides the chromium, magnesium, and NAC that we just mentioned: vitamins B6, B12, and C; calcium; coenzyme Q10; glutathione; folinic acid; omega-3, including alpha-lipoic acid; selenium, and zinc.

L-Arginine and L-Ornithine

L-arginine and L-ornithine are amino acids that play a special role in sexual function and fertility. They work together inside the body and often come packaged together in supplement formulas. They are best known for stimulating both the release of human growth hormone and the creation of nitric oxide in the body, which is important for good blood flow. Naturally, good blood flow supports good sexual function.

In men, L-arginine works as a natural alternative to Viagra. If used for two weeks, L-arginine will increase sperm count and motility by 250 percent. In women, L-arginine causes increased cervical secretions and mucus during the ovulatory phase, and the increase in blood flow leads to enhanced sexual arousal. In one study, women who had failed to conceive for six months to three years began supplementing with L-arginine. By the end of the study, 33 percent of them were pregnant.

L-ornithine is a nonessential amino acid that's made during the breakdown of L-arginine in the body. It serves to build muscle, reduce body fat, increase human growth hormone levels, and boost energy. Also, too much L-arginine can be damaging. L-ornithine does a great job of regulating L-arginine and nitric oxide inside the body.

The body can't use L-arginine and L-ornithine very well if they're taken with lots of sugar.

The Truth about Oral Contraceptives

The use of oral contraceptives ("the Pill") interferes with the body's natural chemistry and hormone levels. It also promotes mineral imbalance in a mother and can even harm the babies that are conceived after a woman stops using the Pill.

The evidence supporting the harmful side effects of oral contraceptives is overwhelming. Aspiring mothers who used the Pill in the past have a higher risk of miscarriage, and since the Pill compromises the immune system, these women are more likely to develop food allergies. Children born to mothers who just stopped taking the Pill are more prone to birthmarks, congenital heart anomalies, skeletal abnormalities, cleft palate, neural tube defects, spina bifida, reduced IQ, and learning difficulties like dyslexia and ADHD. We recommend you give your body as much time as possible without birth control pills before starting a family, at least six months if possible.

Oral contraceptives work by deliberately interfering with a woman's natural hormone system to prevent pregnancy. Oral contraceptives usually contain synthetic versions of the hormones estrogen and progesterone. A healthy woman's levels of natural estrogen and progesterone rise and fall during her menstrual cycle, with higher concentrations occurring toward the end of her cycle.

When a woman becomes pregnant, her estrogen and progesterone levels remain high throughout the pregnancy. This prevents the ovaries from preparing to release another egg. Oral contraceptives work by keeping estrogen and progesterone levels high constantly, confusing the body into thinking it's pregnant all the time. Originally, oral contraceptives contained estrogen only, but this led to irregular bleeding. Progesterone was added to the pill, resulting in the commonly prescribed combination pills, which mostly solved the irregular bleeding issue.

When a woman is taking oral contraceptives, normal menstruation is completely suspended, including ovulatory cycles and bleeding. Contrary to the common myth that the Pill regulates a woman's period "like clockwork," the bleeding that women experience when they stop taking the Pill for a few days each month is *not* normal menstrual bleeding—it is withdrawal bleeding that frequently involves painful cramps and an inflammation response due to prostaglandin release.

Mineral imbalance is a common result of oral contraceptive use. Zinc and manganese deficiency and excess copper levels are characteristic.

As a pregnancy goes on, these mineral imbalances typically get worse. The consequences can include problems during gestation, postpartum depression, and lactation. Zinc deficiency coupled with excess copper can lead to premature birth. Severe manganese and zinc deficiency have been found to eliminate maternal instinct completely in laboratory rats: the normal loving attention that a mother rat displayed toward her pups was absent.

Postpartum depression makes the mineral imbalance even worse, interfering with the body's use of chromium, magnesium, manganese, iron, and iodine and disrupting the metabolism of vitamins B and C. Children of mothers who had these imbalances during pregnancy have displayed difficulties with sexual development. If you've used the Pill and you're going to get your mineral levels tested, pay careful attention to copper, manganese, and zinc.

Another high-risk contraceptive method is the intrauterine device, also known as the coil or the IUD. The coil is a device that a doctor inserts into the womb. It is usually made of toxic substances like plastic, copper, or plastic-coated copper. Its continual presence in the womb prevents pregnancy most of the time, but it's been known to cause extreme complications. Cramping, pain, ectopic pregnancy, spontaneous abortion, uterine bleeding, blood poisoning, bowel obstruction, cervical infection, pelvic infection, infection of the fallopian tubes, dysplasia, cancer of the uterus, perforation of the uterus, and cases in which the device became embedded in the uterus have all been observed. It's a formidable list!

The bottom line is that using any contraceptive method other than the diaphragm, the condom, or the rhythm method can have serious consequences. Even many condoms are made of toxic materials, so take care in selecting a safe brand.

No matter what your doctor or health-care practitioner tells you, oral contraceptives are unhealthy and pose significant health risks. If you're using them, we recommend stopping and then getting your mineral levels tested by a holistic physician. If you've used oral contraceptives in the past, getting a mineral-levels test is important for general health even if you're not planning a pregnancy right away.

The Importance of a Healthy Thyroid

A healthy thyroid is key to a healthy pregnancy. The thyroid, an important component of the endocrine system, is located in the throat area. It sends messages throughout the body about a variety of bodily functions, especially metabolism. Although thyroid disorders include both hypothyroidism (underactive thyroid) and hyperthyroidism (overactive thyroid), hypothyroidism is by far the more common disorder. The symptoms include one or more of the following: fatigue, weakness, weight gain and difficulty losing weight, coarse and dry hair, dry and pale skin, hair loss, cold intolerance (you feel cold in climates in which others are comfortable), muscle cramps and aches, constipation, depression, irritability, memory loss, decreased libido, and an abnormal mentrual cycle. Unfortunately, many of these symptoms are also associated with pregnancy, and the cause can be confusing for doctor and patient alike.

In many cases, a lack of the nutrients required to produce the thyroid hormones T3 and T4 contribute to hypothyroidism. Supplementing with iodine and L-tyrosine can help a lot. Hypothyroidism can also occur as the result of an inflamed thyroid gland (a goiter), which renders much of the gland incapable of producing thyroid hormones. It can also occur if you have an autoimmune disorder in which you produce antibodies that attack the thyroid gland or if the thyroid gland has been removed altogether.

If you haven't had your thyroid level tested recently, we highly recommend getting it checked by a holistic or an antiaging physician. After our first child was born, Lana got her thyroid level tested and discovered she had mild hypothyroidism. Before getting pregnant with our second child, she had her thyroid level corrected.

Working with a holistic or an antiaging physician is key. Many allopathic (conventional Western medical) doctors will test only TSH, which can be normal even if the important thyroid hormones—T3 and T4—are out of range. Even though only a few people have overt hypothyroidism, many people have "subclinical" hypothyroidism, which doesn't show up on the conventional test but is still not healthy and may even cause unpleasant symptoms. Holistic and antiaging doctors usually know that "fine" isn't "great," and they'll work with you to optimize the levels of the thyroid hormones T3 and T4.

Research indicates that a baby's well-being and intelligence are related to the mother's thyroid health. Overt and subclinical hypothyroidism and hyperthyroidism have been linked to miscarriage, premature birth, and preeclampsia. Researchers in Maine who observed more than twenty-five thousand women found that 19 percent of the children born to mothers with untreated hypothyroidism had an IQ below 85, while only 5 percent of mothers with healthy thyroid levels had children with such a low IQ. People with an IQ of 85 or below find school and general life tasks to be more difficult than most other people do.

Overall, we found ourselves to be much healthier and happier after we had our thyroid levels corrected. There's some debate about the safety of taking thyroid hormones during pregnancy. Nonetheless, pregnancy is when thyroid problems are more common than usual. It's our position that hypothyroidism is a greater risk than supplementing with bioidentical thyroid hormones during pregnancy. If you're concerned about the risks of taking thyroid hormones during pregnancy, you can always optimize your thyroid level before getting pregnant and then reduce the thyroid hormones before you conceive. If you need to stay on thyroid supplementation during pregnancy, as Lana did with our second child, you should have your thyroid levels checked regularly.

Sickness and Sexually Transmitted Diseases

Diseases, especially sexually transmitted diseases (STDs), can compromise fertility and harm your baby. Making sure that both the father and the mother are free of diseases, especially STDs, well before conceiving is essential to having the healthiest baby possible. The most common diseases to check for are AIDS, hepatitis B, gardnerella (a vaginal infection), mumps, listeriosis, influenza, genitourinary infection, urinary tract infection, *Candida* overgrowth, chlamydia, mycoplasma (in the cervical mucus), gonorrhea, herpes, syphilis, and pelvic inflammatory disease. When you're planning for a pregnancy, it's best for both partners to get a complete genitourinary examination, even if you both believe that you don't have anything. This is especially true if you're having difficulty conceiving.

Fertility Treatment: Not Just for Women

We all know that babies begin when a sperm meets an egg. When people think of fertility treatment, they tend to focus on making healthy eggs without giving much thought to making healthy sperm. To have the healthiest baby possible, it makes sense to focus on both. Not only do we want to have healthy eggs and an ideal womb environment, we also want to ensure that the sperm are healthy and well formed. Building above-average babies starts with above-average eggs and above-average sperm.

Although the mother's job is considerable and gets the most attention, the father has two key responsibilities that, if neglected, can work strongly against any effort the mother makes:

1. Having high sperm quality. Sperm quality can be improved the same way that the mother improves her fertility and womb environment: through proper nutrition, detoxification, and psychological and emotional well-being.

2. Providing emotional support for his mate while she's pregnant and vulnerable. He needs to take action to create a stable environment, reduce her stress level, and show unconditional love. He's responsible for making sure that the fear-of-loss mechanism in her brain is triggered as few times as possible during pregnancy. Reducing the mother's fear limits the baby's exposure to cortisol and epinephrine, the hormones that send him or her into a defensive neural program and take energy away from growth.

There are three things that determine sperm quality: count, motility, and morphology. A normal *count* is at least twenty million sperm per milliliter. *Motility* is the number of sperm making functional use of their flagella and moving forward, or "swimming." At least 50 percent should display progressive movement. *Morphology* concerns the shape of the sperm. At least 14 percent of the sperm should be formed normally, which means that the sperm cell does not have an unusually large head, does not have two heads, has healthy cell proportions, and displays progressive motility.

For any couple reading this book, maintaining good sperm quality in the male will be quite convenient—all of the recommendations we make for women concerning diet, detoxification, and psychological and emotional well-being also boost sperm quality in men. Aspiring fathers and mothers who have followed our program have felt so much better from it that soon after they began, they didn't view it as a chore anymore. Also, by sticking to the program, the man supports the woman and helps her to follow it.

There are a few supplements that boost sperm quality: zinc, acetyl-L-carnitine, coenzyme Q10, lycopene, and vitamins C, E, and B12.

Zinc is a key supplement for male fertility. The testes and the prostate naturally contain high levels of zinc, and a zinc deficiency can lead to reduced testosterone levels. Supplementing with zinc has been found to improve sperm quality in infertile men: taking 250 milligrams of zinc twice daily for three months significantly improved sperm count, progressive motility, and fertilizing capacity while reducing the presence of sperm-fighting antibodies.

The acetyl-L-carnitine level has been shown to be lower in infertile men than in fertile men. In the study, the treatment group received acetyl-L-carnitine and showed significantly improved mobile sperm counts compared to the control group. Carnitines appear to be necessary for the function of sperm cells, and supplementation with acetyl-L-carnitine is effective at raising the level.

As a mitochondrial factor involved in energy metabolism, coenzyme Q10 protects sperm from oxidative stress. Infertile men who were given one hundred milligrams of coenzyme Q10 twice a day for six months showed a significant rise in sperm motility, from 9 to 16 percent. When the men stopped taking coenzyme Q10, their semen profiles returned to the 9 percent baseline level two months later.

Lycopene is an antioxidant found in high concentration in the testes and the seminal plasma. In one study, twenty infertile men took two thousand micrograms of lycopene twice a day for three months. As a result, 66 percent showed an improvement in sperm count, 53 percent had improved progressive motility, and 46 percent showed improvement in sperm morphology.

Vitamin C protects sperm from oxidative damage and is especially helpful for sperm quality in smokers and men with agglutination, a problem with semen consistency.

The herb ginkgo biloba has been shown to support blood flow and erectile function. L-arginine and L-ornithine, which we discussed earlier, strongly support male sexual function and fertility as well.

Alcohol, tobacco, and excessive caffeine—all commonly consumed by men—are just as harmful for sperm and male fertility as they are for pregnant women and fetuses. Alcohol abuse lowers the testosterone level, shrinks the testes, creates difficulty in achieving and sustaining an erection, and slows sperm production. One Danish study found that miscarriage was more frequent among women whose partners had two or more alcoholic drinks per day during the month before conception. California researchers found that couples in which the male partner routinely drank alcohol were less likely to have a successful pregnancy than couples in which the male didn't drink alcohol.

The father's age is also a factor. Researchers in Israel sifted through medical records and discovered that children born to fathers over forty years of age were six times more likely to have autism, and children of fathers over fifty years of age were nine times more likely. One of many possible explanations for the dramatic increase in the rate of autism in the United States is that the rate of men over forty who are fathering children has increased by about 40 percent since 1980. Simultaneously, men under thirty are having 21 percent fewer children since 1980.

The same researchers linked older fathers to an increased rate of birth defects, cleft palate, water on the brain, dwarfism, miscarriage, "decreased intellectual capacity," and schizophrenia. Like the rate of autism, the rates of schizophrenia and bipolar disorder in children also increased with a father's age.

Other studies mention that older fathers may contribute to prostate or other cancer in their children. Other disorders linked to the father's age are progeria (rapid premature aging) and Marfan syndrome (strangely long arms, legs, and fingers, along with heart defects). Overall, the data suggest that the father's health is just as important as the mother's health for a successful pregnancy. For example, the rates of a forty-year-old man having a child with schizophrenia and a forty-year-old woman having a child with Down syndrome are the same.

We're not presenting this information to suggest that older men refrain from having children. When we did our own research, age was an important consideration for us because Lana was almost forty years old. Yet even though Dave was only thirty-four when we had our first child, he took just as many precautions as Lana did. We know that there's a higher risk of things going wrong for older parents and that this risk increases with age—there's no dispute about that in the scientific community.

Because of this, we do believe that like older aspiring mothers, older aspiring fathers owe it to themselves, their partners, and their children to take appropriate steps to counteract the higher risk that they face. After careful research, we believe that we present the best techniques for reducing risk that are available today. These include proper diet and supplementation, detoxification, and emotional support for mothers and fathers. And we recommend that like aspiring mothers, aspiring fathers start on this regimen six months before the couple plans to conceive.

Sex for Pregnancy

The most fertile sexual positions are those that stimulate orgasm in the woman. Orgasm isn't necessary for a woman to become pregnant, but it does help pull sperm toward the egg. For a couple trying to get pregnant, the man's goal should be to satisfy the woman and bring her to climax. Finishing sex in the missionary position can help with conception, because this position is conducive to releasing sperm deep into the vagina.

After sex, the woman can put a pillow under her hips to elevate them and give gravity a chance to help sperm and egg meet. Using a lubricant can help a lot and can take pressure off the woman to perform sexually. Pre-Seed is a safe, nontoxic lubricant that won't harm sperm or the womb environment.

7

Your Prenatal Supplement Regimen

Six months before pregnancy is an ideal time to start a supplement regimen. This will help your body to detoxify, build up reserves, and achieve greater health and vitality in preparation for pregnancy.

The supplements we took before pregnancy cost about three hundred dollars per month because both of us were taking large amounts of high-quality brands. Depending on your choices, it's possible to keep your prepregnancy supplement bill to under one hundred dollars per month. Even this isn't cheap, but we've found it to be an excellent investment, considering the reduced health risk and the lifelong health benefits you and your kids will gain. As with many products, when it comes to dietary supplements, you usually get what you pay for, although there are some very expensive, and useless, supplements. And supplements are most expensive when they don't work, no matter what you paid for them.

Some nutrients work best when taken on an empty stomach, and some work best when taken with food. Some are ideal in the morning, and some work best at night. For this reason, Lana took some supplements when she woke up, some when she ate, and some before she went to bed. Many supplements do not stay in your system for more than eight to twelve hours, so taking them twice a day will keep your level of nutrition more even during the vital period that your baby is growing in your womb. As we discuss each nutrient separately, we'll explain how it is best used.

Before buying and using nutritional supplements, we suggest that you work with an alternative or holistic doctor or health-care practitioner to measure your vitamin and mineral levels and correct deficiencies or excesses. The central principle to supplementation is realizing that your body is individual and therefore biochemically different from other people's bodies, which means there's no one-size-fits-all supplement regimen that will be best for everyone. Some people may need many times the FDA's recommended daily intake of a particular nutrient. Working with a holistic physician is best, because the physician can help you to determine your individual needs. Our suggestions are general guidelines, but your needs are specific, so please do work with a doctor.

How to Tell if a Supplement Is Useful and Safe

A key element of supplementation is making sure you buy supplements that are *bioavailable*, that your body can absorb and use. You can test absorbability by taking an individual tablet or capsule and placing it in a glass of white vinegar heated to ninety-nine degrees Fahrenheit. This simulates the stomach environment rather well. If the tablet or capsule dissolves within thirty minutes, your body is probably absorbing a good amount of the supplement. If the tablet or capsule doesn't dissolve, the supplement is a waste of money, because it's likely to move through your gastrointestinal tract with minimal absorption. So if the supplement doesn't dissolve, it's time to find a new brand. You'll find that the supplements that dissolve best are often capsules and not tablets. We've tested all the brands we recommend on www.betterbabybook.com/supplements, and we use them ourselves.

When evaluating supplement brands, we always read the label to see if the inactive ingredients (the binders) are harmful or make the supplement hard for the body to use. Ideally, your supplements will be in capsules, so the only ingredient should be the nutrient blend itself, the gelatin capsule or vegetarian capsule material (listed as MHCP), and magnesium stearate (a safe binder). Many cheap and popular supplements, especially those sold in drugstores and by large vitamin chains, contain added sugar, starch, salt, wheat, gluten, corn, colorings like titanium dioxide, dairy products or casein, flavoring, or preservatives. The same principles for buying food apply to buying supplements: if you see any ingredient you don't recognize, find out what the ingredient is before buying and trying.

Just like food, supplements can go bad or get moldy. Most supplements are best stored in a cool, dry, dark place. If a supplement can go bad, we store it in the refrigerator when appropriate.

Any time you take a supplement, it's best to evaluate its interactions with foods, other supplements, or drugs. This goes especially for herbs. If you're not sure about a particular combination, we suggest checking with a holistic physician, a midwife, or an herbalist. As health experts, we knew the things that we did were safe.

The Myth of *a* Prenatal Supplement

Most pregnant women get *a* prenatal supplement from their physicians and assume they're covered. They are, if the goal is to avoid the diseases caused only by extreme nutritional deficiency, like rickets. The acute deficiencies that cause these diseases aren't a problem in most Western countries, however. So even though a prenatal supplement will surely help, most pregnant women need far more than what's contained in one tablet or capsule for their pregnancies to go as well as possible. One prenatal a day isn't likely to give your child the best start he or she can have.

Nonetheless, people are led to believe that if a woman takes a single one-a-day prenatal supplement, her fetus will be protected from birth defects and her womb will be an optimal developmental environment. This is a marketing lie. Most prenatal supplements don't contain near the amount of nutrients a pregnant woman needs. In fact, we found that most prenatal supplements aren't much more than basic multivitamins that contain extra folic acid. The size of most prenatal supplements isn't even large enough to contain just the calcium and magnesium alone that a pregnant woman needs, not to mention everything else. Also, many prenatal supplements are glorified candy loaded with sugar and toxins. They're dyed with artificial coloring and contain dangerous binding agents.

Even though prenatals aren't enough, if you do only one thing we recommend in this chapter, take a high-quality food-based prenatal supplement in conjunction with a multivitamin. Depending on the brand and the potency, three to five prenatal capsules per day in addition to five to seven multivitamin capsules is usually ideal. Our website lists high-strength, high-quality prenatals and multivitamins that have no additives or ingredients known to be harmful to a fetus at normal doses. As always, consult with a holistic physician if you don't know what to do.

Prenatal supplements are also helpful when you're trying to conceive. The same factors that promote a healthy pregnancy promote fertility. This is even more important for women who have just stopped taking oral contraceptives. As we mentioned in the previous chapter, women who take oral contraceptives often have lower levels of essential vitamins and minerals, including B2, B6, vitamin C, folate, and zinc. Deficiencies in these nutrients invite problems, which we discuss in the following sections.

Multivitamins

Multivitamins are an effective way to cover your bases and make sure you aren't dangerously deficient in any essential vitamin or mineral. A good multivitamin will be a nonsynthetic food-based capsule, tablet, or liquid that contains carotenoids; B complex; vitamins C, D, E, and K; and a good mix of minerals and fatty acids in a form useful to the body.

Before and during pregnancy, we used multivitamins as general support for our specialized supplements for fetal brain development and function, birth-defect prevention, and prevention of a premature delivery. We took the multivitamins, because there's little point to high-end, targeted supplementation without covering the body's basic needs.

As a result of marketing, many people believe the lie that one or two multivitamins a day provides your body with all of the nutrients you need. Many of these recommended daily doses are based on the

FDA's recommended daily intake figures. Studies have proven some of the FDA's figures to be woefully inadequate, however, especially for vitamin D3. During pregnancy, of course, the requirements are even higher. Lana took seven to nine multivitamin tablets a day during both pregnancies. "One a day" is good for marketing, but not for nutrition!

In the rest of this chapter we cover the supplements that act to prevent miscarriage and protect your baby from common birth defects. If you take no others, these are the supplements you'll want to take for three to six months before getting pregnant to build up healthy levels. We recommend working with a holistic physician well before pregnancy to make sure your hormone levels are correct.

Essential Vitamins

The basis of any good supplement regimen begins, of course, with the basic vitamins: A, B, C, D, E, and K.

Vitamin A

Full-form vitamin A (mostly retinyl palmitate) is an ester (a compound formed by the reaction between an acid and an alcohol) that's converted into the alcohol retinol in the small intestine. Your body uses retinol for good vision, gene transcription, and immune function. Vitamin A is also a part of fertility and embryo development. It is yellow and fat-soluble. One of the unique properties of retinyl groups like vitamin A is their ability to absorb light. That's why vitamin A is so important for proper eye function. A deficiency in vitamin A can result in night blindness (the inability to see in low-light conditions). An ongoing deficiency can lead to full blindness.

Vitamin A plays a big role in early fetal development. Giving your baby vitamin A supplements after birth won't compensate for a shortage of vitamin A during critical development stages in the womb. Yellow, orange, and green fruits and vegetables are very rich in vitamin A. Examples of yellow and orange sources are sweet potatoes, carrots, pumpkin, cantaloupe, apricots, papaya, mangoes, and winter squash. Green sources are broccoli and broccoli leaves, kale, spinach, leafy vegetables, collard greens, and peas. Butter from grass-fed cows and free-range eggs are good sources, as well as the livers of cows, pigs, chickens, and turkeys.

Even if you're eating plenty of vitamin A, you can still be deficient in it. That's because vitamin A has to mix with normal dietary fats and zinc to become useful inside your body. Our diet is rich in the fats you need for this. Beef shanks, cashews, almonds, and peas are good sources of zinc, but we recommend taking a good zinc supplement, too.

Vitamin A's Complication

There's a complication with vitamin A that's important to understand: it's easy to have too much, and too much of it spells trouble for both mother and baby. Since vitamin A is fat-soluble, it's hard for your body to eliminate it. Water-soluble vitamins like B and C don't pose this problem (anything water-soluble is easily eliminated). Toxicity from other fat-soluble vitamins (D, E, and K) happens far less often than vitamin A toxicity. It's estimated that more than 75 percent of people in developed nations get too much pre-formed vitamin A.

Vitamin A toxicity causes nausea, jaundice, loss of appetite, blurry vision, drowsiness, and related disorders. If a pregnant woman has too much vitamin A, it's very harmful for her baby: too much vitamin A can disrupt brain cell activity. During organogenesis (the formation of the baby's organs), a fetus is even more susceptible to harm from vitamin A toxicity. Since vitamin A toxicity symptoms are very similar to routine symptoms during pregnancy, it's important to get your vitamin A level checked.

Too much vitamin A is doubly dangerous, because vitamin A competes with vitamin D inside the body. Too much vitamin A deprives the body of D, which is critically important for fetal development. Excess vitamin A has been linked to osteoporosis for this very reason: it blocks D from working with calcium to support proper bone growth and maintenance. At the other extreme, however—if you don't get enough vitamin A—vitamin D will "use up" your vitamin A. A further complication in the relationship is that vitamins A and D actually work together in some tasks that are critical for your baby's development. For instance, A helps D to bind with DNA to promote optimal gene translation.

A Simple Answer for a Complex Situation

This all sounds quite complicated, and it is. Fortunately, there's a simple solution to getting this right: you'll get vitamin A toxicity only if you eat too much *fully formed* vitamin A. This is not likely to happen unless you take too much of a vitamin A supplement or you eat very excessive amounts of liver or liver oils (like cod liver oil).

The food sources of vitamin A listed above actually don't contain much fully formed A; they contain vitamin A *provitamins*, which the body uses to build fully formed vitamins. In this case, the provitamins are carotenoids, which include beta carotene. Your body can use carotenoids to make fully formed retinoid vitamin A only when it needs vitamin A. Eating too many carotenoids is not toxic to you or your baby, although you can develop a yellow-orange skin discoloration if you really eat a lot. If you eat plenty of yellow, orange, and green vegetables with a decent amount of good dietary fats and zinc, your body will make the perfect amount of vitamin A all by itself!

Balancing vitamins A and D is simple if you follow these guidelines:

- Eat green, orange, and yellow vegetables to get the building blocks for vitamin A.

- If your D level is low, supplement with D3 until your level is optimal.

- Don't take fully formed A supplements unless you know you're deficient in vitamin A, and don't eat too much liver or liver oils.

Vitamin B

B vitamins work together and should always be taken together. For this reason, almost all B vitamin supplements come as a B-complex. A good B-complex supplement will consist of the following: B1 (thiamine), B2 (riboflavin), B3 (niacin), B5 (pantothenic acid), B6 (pyridoxine), B7 (biotin), B9 (folate *not* folic acid), and B12 (methylcobalamin or hydroxocobalamin), along with para-amino benzoic acid (PABA). For preventing neural tube defects, vitamins B5, B9, and B12 are the champions.

B5: Pantothenic Acid

Pantothenic acid, or B5, is used to change sugars and fats into energy, and it also plays a role in protein metabolism. B5 facilitates the creation of cholesterol steroids and fatty acids and helps the body use choline and PABA to sustain proper adrenal function and regulation, better enabling the body to withstand stress. It also aids in the creation and growth of antibodies for immune protection.

A deficiency in pantothenic acid leads to a shortage of adrenal hormones and poor adrenal function, low blood sugar and blood pressure, and a shortage of digestive enzymes and slow peristaltic (intestinal) action. The symptoms are indigestion, constipation, food allergies, depression, discontentment, irritability, and, in extreme cases, nausea, vomiting, and insomnia. The chronic stress from exhausted adrenals and the headaches and dizziness that result from low blood sugar are known to harm an unborn baby's central nervous system. In lab animals, a pantothenic acid deficiency is linked to abnormalities in the nervous system, cleft palate, heart defects, club foot, poor myelination (sheathing) of nerve tissue, and miscarriage. Similar effects are suspected in people.

Pantothenic acid is abundant in many foods, especially in organ meats, egg yolks, and green vegetables. Pantothenic acid is water-soluble and nontoxic, so we recommend taking at least an additional ten milligrams per day during pregnancy to make sure you have enough. Pantothenic acid will protect your baby, and Lana found that it eased the daily stresses of pregnancy.

Folate: The Right Form of Folic Acid

For a long time women of childbearing age have been advised to supplement with folic acid, or B9, to prevent neural tube defects in their children. This practice has reduced neural tube defect prevalence by 50 to 70 percent. But many people don't know that folic acid is the just the beginning of what you can do to protect your baby, and that the commonly used form isn't the right one.

Epigenetics has taught us that the best times to prevent miscarriage and birth defects are before pregnancy and immediately after conception. Early miscarriage may result from a state of poor nutrition or hormonal imbalance immediately preceding conception. Many serious birth defects originate within the first eight weeks of pregnancy while the baby's organs are forming.

Nearly everyone has heard that pregnant women should take folic acid to prevent birth defects. What they haven't heard is that folic acid is the synthetic form and that only a small percentage of folic acid converts to the active form, which is called *folate* or *folinic acid* (sometimes marketed as tetrahydorfolate or 5-MTHF). To make matters worse, 60 percent of people have genes that reduce their ability to convert folic acid into the active form. We need the active form of folate to synthesize, repair, and express DNA—all essential processes for using epigenetics to improve your baby's lifelong health.

Folate is used to form red blood cells in bone marrow, where it also helps to make antibodies by using sugars and amino acids. Folate works with vitamin B12 in the formation of hemoglobin and is essential for zinc metabolism. It's a fundamental ingredient to good health and plays a crucial role in pregnancy, because a mother's body needs a lot of it to share with her baby.

The benefits of taking folate during pregnancy have been widely publicized, and it's included (as the synthetic form, folic acid) in most prenatal supplements. Nonetheless, a deficiency is common during pregnancy. A mother's deficiency in folate can lead to fetal abnormalities like cleft palate, harelip, deformed limbs, neural tube defects like spina bifida, skeletal deformities, lung and kidney underdevelopment, cataracts, brain deformities, and anemia. Underdevelopment of the heart, diaphragm, urogenital system, blood vessels, adrenals, and eyes can also result.

Supplementing with *folinic* acid especially helps to prevent fetal abnormalities relating to neural tube defects. Studies suggest that women who supplement with folate during the month of conception and the first eight to ten weeks after conception are less likely to have a malformed baby. We recommend taking 800 micrograms per day. Good sources of the active form of folate are green leafy vegetables, organ meats, root vegetables, and nuts.

Folinic acid supplements are very affordable, and it's worth spending about five dollars more a month to get this form instead of plain folic acid. When taken as a supplement, synthetic folic acid begins to accumulate in the bloodstream at just 400 micrograms per day. This means it isn't being processed by the body.

B12: A Versatile Nutrient

B12 has many uses. It is part of the production and regeneration of red blood cells and the general metabolic function of proteins, carbohydrates, and fats. It's a key component of a certain sequence of enzyme reactions known as the Krebs cycle. B12 also aids the body in the use of iron, combines with folic acid to form choline, and is a component in the formation of RNA and DNA.

A deficiency in B12 is dangerous. A mild deficiency can lead to pernicious anemia, nerve degeneration, a sore mouth and tongue, and brain damage. A severe deficiency can lead to deterioration of the spinal cord and eventually paralysis. B12's large role in nerve function underscores its importance in the proper development of your baby's neural tube and nervous system.

Research links a low B12 level with an increased risk of neural tube defects (they accounted for preexisting folate levels). They noticed that B12 was metabolically related to folate and that previous studies had also found mothers of children with neural tube defects to be low in B12. The study concluded that women should have B12 levels over 300 nanograms per liter (221 picomoles per liter) before becoming pregnant.

Good food sources of B12 are organ meats, eggs, dulse and kelp (types of seaweed), and spirulina. If you supplement with B-complex, it's best to take it with vitamin C and with meals. Cyanocobalamin is the most popular form of B12, but the body doesn't absorb it very well. When looking for a quality B12 supplement that your body will easily absorb and use, look for the B12 ingredient to be methylcobalamin or hydroxocobalamin. Vitamin B12 is almost always found in foods made from animal products, so if you're a vegan, it's even more important to find a good B12 supplement.

Vitamin C

Vitamin C (ascorbic acid) is a potent antioxidant that plays a central role in collagen synthesis. Collagen is a big part of our blood vessels, tendons, ligaments, and bones. Vitamin C keeps the body resistant to penetration by intruders like viruses, toxins, or dangerous drugs; it promotes healing after infection, injury, or surgery and keeps the capillary walls in good form; and it helps the body to absorb and use iron, preventing anemia. As an ingredient of the neurotransmitter norepinephrine, vitamin C is important for mental health, and as an ingredient in carnitine, it supports metabolism and a healthy energy level.

A deficiency in vitamin C can result in scurvy, dandruff, hemorrhaging, spontaneous bleeding, infection, easily broken bones, and, most important for our purpose here, miscarriage. Good food sources of vitamin C are citrus fruits, tomatoes, broccoli and other green vegetables (including parsley), strawberries, apples, pears, carrots, and cauliflower. Vitamin C is water-soluble and is lost in storage in the body, so it's important to take a good supplement or eat foods rich in vitamin C regularly. Vitamin C is most useful to the body when it's taken with other vitamins and minerals, bioflavonoids, calcium, and magnesium, so the best time to take it is with a meal.

Vitamin D

Vitamin D-3 (cholecalciferol) is actually not a vitamin, it's a prohormone. Prohormones are building blocks of fully formed bioactive hormones. When a person is exposed to sunlight, vitamin D is produced naturally in the skin and the eyes. It can also be taken effectively as a supplement. Much of what we know about vitamin D comes from John Cannell, a doctor who is the head of the Vitamin D Council in San Luis Obispo, California. For years he has published world-class research on the involvement of vitamin D deficiency in a wide range of health problems.

Vitamin D has the following functions inside the body:

- It is central to brain and nervous system function and the prevention of multiple sclerosis.

- It is central to fertility and the prevention of breast, uterine, colon and ovarian cancers.

- It boosts the immune system by increasing the natural production of antibiotic and antiviral mechanisms inside the body, which prevents short-term infections like influenza and colds.

- It detoxifies the brain and body of heavy metals like mercury.

- It helps the body to bind and eliminate mycotoxins.

- It aids in the correct translation of more than two thousand genes (nearly 10 percent of your genes).

- It reduces the severity of the body's (autoimmune) attacks on its own tissues.

The detoxifying benefits make vitamin D as important for prospective fathers as for expecting mothers. When a man deficient in vitamin D ingests toxins, they cause oxidative damage that can result in genetic mutations (genetic damage) in sperm. These mutations can lead to autism in children.

In a recent study, vitamin D proved so important for fetal nervous system and cognition development that even mothers who consumed more mercury-contaminated fish (fish naturally has some vitamin D) had babies with higher than average cognition. That is, vitamin D is so beneficial for a developing fetus that it counteracted the harmful effects of toxic mercury to produce a net benefit.

Another study proved that this net effect was not a result of the omega-3 fatty acids in the fish. Yet another concluded that mothers who consumed less mercury-contaminated fish during pregnancy had babies who exhibited more autistic symptoms than the babies of mothers who consumed more mercury-containing fish. Of course, eating mercury-free fish rich in vitamin D would be a better option, and fortunately it's an option we still have.

Vitamin D Deficiency and Autism

Research suggests that a vitamin D deficiency contributes to autism. This makes sense if autism is a neuroinflammatory condition, because vitamin D protects the body from neurotoxins. Consider these facts:

- Autism is more common in cloudy, rainy regions.

- People with darker skin have a higher rate of autism than people with lighter skin. Darker skin protects a person from ultraviolet exposure better than lighter skin does, but it also causes a person to make less vitamin D from a given level of sun exposure than a person with lighter skin would make.

- Autism is more common in the northern United States than in the southern part of the country. There is less direct sun exposure in the northern regions.

- Autism is more common in urban regions, where the lifestyle is more indoors, than in rural regions, where an outdoor lifestyle is common.

- Bone abnormalities are more common in autistic children than they are in nonautistic children. The abnormalities often resemble mild cases of chronic rickets, a bone disorder resulting from a vitamin D deficiency.

Other Risks of Vitamin D Deficiency

Vitamin D deficiency in a mother has been linked to a number of risks related to her pregnancy and the health of her child. A vitamin D deficiency is surely dangerous for a pregnant woman, but irreversible damage may be done to her child in utero. Vitamin D is required for proper development during critical development stages, so its absence can have lasting effects that will not be reversed with vitamin D supplements after birth. Some of the effects may not become evident until the child is in his or her thirties.

Vitamin D deficiency has been linked to the following risks in mother and child:

Risks for Mother

- Bacterial vaginitis (twice as likely).
- Caesarian section (four times as likely).
- Gestational diabetes (three times as likely).
- Preeclampsia (five times as likely).
- Premature birth.

Risks for Baby

- Asthma (vitamin D is critical to fetal lung development).
- Cavities in young children.
- Certain brain tumors and epilepsy—correlated with winter births, when a mother's vitamin D level is naturally lower.

- Infant heart failure.

- Lower respiratory tract infections in infants.

- Schizophrenia (the risk increases dramatically, and the rates have increased in recent years). Factors associated with increased rates are prenatal infection, omega-3 deficiency, and vitamin D deficiency.

- Seizures from hypocalcemia (calcium deficiency).

- Sepsis in premature infants.

- Weak bones later in life.

Optimizing Your D Level

You should supplement with D to have the best possible pregnancy. Ideally, you should start well before pregnancy to build up your levels. Once a fetus has been exposed to neurotoxins like mercury with no vitamin D to protect it, it can sometimes be too late to reverse the damage. We believe that supplying the child with appropriate amounts of vitamin D after birth will undoubtedly improve his or her health, but it's never been observed to make up for the damage done from a vitamin D deficiency during critical development stages in the womb.

The first step is to have a 25-hydroxy vitamin D (known as a 25-OH-D) blood test done. (The 1.25-dihydroxy vitamin D test that many physicians use is ineffective.) This test is available for purchase without a doctor's prescription. If you're working with a doctor's office, be sure to ask for a copy of your test results. Your vitamin D level should be between 50 and 80 nanograms per milliliter. If it's lower than that, don't be surprised. Less than 5 percent of Americans are in this ideal range. If you're below 50 nanograms per milliliter, any little bit of D the body gets is instantly used, and there is no reserve.

In November 2008, the American Academy of Pediatrics advised obstetric health-care professionals nationwide to administer 25-OH-D tests to their patients and recommend supplementation to patients with levels below 32 nanograms per milliliter. Although that level might be enough, we made sure that both of our levels were around 80 nanograms per milliliter before we conceived.

If your vitamin D level is sufficient and you choose not to supplement it, we recommend monitoring your level throughout pregnancy to make sure it doesn't fall out of range (especially in the winter). If the test shows that you're deficient, which D supplement should you buy and how much should you take?

In a 2008 study led by the aforementioned Dr. Cannell of the Vitamin D Council, seventeen experts agreed that children need 1,000 international units for every twenty-five pounds of body weight, and pregnant and lactating women need 5,000 to 7,000 international units per day. This means that the minuscule amount of vitamin D contained in ordinary prenatal vitamins (as little as 400 to 600 international units) is woefully inadequate.

A 2006 study followed pregnant women taking 400, 2,000, and 4,000 international units per day. It found that even though 4,000 was a safe amount, it wasn't enough, because the newborns' vitamin D blood levels were only 27 nanograms per milliliter; 40 is ideal. The women who were taking 2,000 units per day had more infections than the women who were taking 4,000 units, and the women who were taking only 400 units per day had twice as many pregnancy complications as the women who were taking 4,000 units per day.

A number of companies now manufacture pharmaceutical-grade vitamin D, and it's usually cheap. Be sure to get vitamin D3 (cholecalciferol), which is the form of vitamin D that your body makes in sunlight. Vitamin D2 (ergocalciferol) is a synthetic vitamin D that has different effects inside the body than D3 does. Most vitamin D that's added to milk is D2, not D3, so vitamin D–enriched milk is not an effective supplement.

Maintaining a vitamin D sufficiency in your baby after birth is equally important. One study found that babies who took in more than 2,000 international units of vitamin D every day were 80 percent less likely to contract type 1 diabetes. Children who are deficient in vitamin D are six times more likely to have asthma than children who take vitamin D supplements.

Vitamin E

Vitamin E is a family of oil-soluble antioxidants called *tocopherols*. Vitamin E prevents the oxidation of vitamin A and is required for the proper use of essential fatty acids and selenium. It also prevents scarring after burns, seals abrasions, and possibly helps to reverse congenital heart defects in infants when it is given very early in the baby's life. A vitamin E deficiency can lead to anemia, an enlarged prostate gland, premature aging, liver and kidney damage, and muscular degeneration.

Vitamin E helps to ease labor pains by strengthening the abdominal muscles. It's often used in prolonged labor because weak muscles can lead to problems for the baby, who can become starved of oxygen during that time. Good food sources of vitamin E are healthy cold-pressed oils, egg yolks, green leafy vegetables, and avocados. Vitamin E is most useful to the body when taken at mealtime with vitamins A, B complex, and C and essential fatty acids, manganese, and selenium.

Vitamin K

Vitamin K is a group of oil-soluble vitamin structures that are typically made by probiotic flora in a healthy GI tract. It is essential for blood clotting, so when a woman goes into labor, vitamin K is sometimes injected to control bleeding. We do not recommend this if you can avoid it—one study linked these injections to childhood leukemia.

If a woman is healthy and eats plenty of green leafy vegetables, she most likely has enough stored vitamin K and its building blocks for a healthy pregnancy. Research has found that if a mother is deficient in vitamin K, her baby is at higher risk for birth defects, including cardiac dysfunction, craniofacial abnormalities, a flat nasal bridge, growth and learning disorders, microcephaly (an abnormally small head), and neural tube defects. To make sure Lana had sufficient vitamin K, she took the right probiotics and a very small amount of the vitamin itself.

Essential Minerals

Essential mineral supplements help to ensure that your body is performing correctly and supporting your baby's growth to its greatest potential. The most important minerals are calcium, chromium, cobalt, copper, iodine, iron, magnesium, manganese, nickel, phosphorous, potassium, selenium, vanadium, and zinc.

Essential minerals work together and with other vitamins and nutrients, so it's best to take them with a meal. Before starting a mineral supplement regimen, we recommend seeing a holistic physician and having your mineral levels checked. Hair mineral analysis is very effective. Go to www.betterbabybook.com/minerals for a complete description of each mineral, what it does inside the body, the best way to supplement with it, and a list of foods that contain it.

Here we will discuss iron and iodine, two minerals that are most important for pregnancy, although you should take a broad spectrum multi-mineral supplement with extra magnesium, too.

Iron

The body needs iron to make hemoglobin, the molecule that carries oxygen in the blood. Oxygen is essential for life. Without iron to make hemoglobin, breathing wouldn't do you any good—the oxygen you breathed wouldn't reach any of the places in your body that need it. Iron helps the body to support resistance to infection and is central to respiratory function and detoxification.

Pregnant women need lots of iron, because their red blood cell count increases by 30 percent during pregnancy. Lots of iron maintains a healthy hemoglobin concentration during this blood increase. Iron isn't absorbed well without vitamin C (ascorbic acid). If iron is taken by itself without vitamin C, it can lower the body's supply of other key minerals.

In the early stages of pregnancy, women often become thirsty and drink lots of water. That water is taken to the placenta and used to make the amniotic fluid, but for a short period the blood is diluted, and some women may be diagnosed with iron deficiency. Be sure not to take too much iron under these circumstances (especially without vitamin C)—you may actually *have* plenty of iron! Even a sixty-milligram iron supplement might be too much. At the other extreme, an iron deficiency can be devastating for a fetus. Iron must be kept in proper balance. Work with your ob-gyn or nutritionist to test your levels.

When you're supplementing with iron, it's best to use iron-rich foods (organic iron) rather than tablet or capsule supplement products.

Most supplements contain inorganic iron, which is difficult for the body to absorb. If you choose to use a supplement, studies suggest that organic elemental iron is more effective than the inorganic forms. Using iron-rich foods is also better than iron supplements, because the foods contain plenty of other minerals as well. This prevents a situation in which high amounts of isolated iron are depleting your body of other important minerals.

Good iron sources are almonds, egg yolks, kelp, parsley, beef from grass-fed cows, and green leafy vegetables. Eating a poached egg (with runny yolk) and taking vitamin C at the same time is a great way to boost your iron level.

Iodine

Iodine is a trace mineral that's essential for life. It plays a key role in thyroid function, which regulates metabolism. The thyroid itself is regulated by the thyroid hormones triiodothyronine (T3) and thyroxine (T4), both of which are composed of more than 50 percent iodine. A chronic iodine deficiency leads to slow metabolism and hypothyroidism, which manifests as fatigue, weight gain, depression, dry skin, low body temperature, loss of interest in sex, anorexia, slow pulse, high cholesterol, and sometimes heart disease and cancer. Severe iodine deficiency results in goiter, a swelling of the thyroid gland. Iodine is toxic in high quantities and is deadly in quantities over three grams. An overdose can result in abnormal growth of the thyroid glands, which leads to many of the same symptoms as iodine deficiency.

Hypothyroidism during pregnancy can lead to cretinism in children. Cretinism is a congenital disease that can result in mental and physical retardation. The World Health Organization names iodine deficiency as the leading cause of brain damage in the world today.

Iodine is also important for the function of the mammary glands and is present in the cervix of healthy women. Iodine is especially important for women, because it modulates the estrogen pathway, helping to keep female reproductive function in good order. Iodine sufficiency promotes healthy breast function, and a deficiency heightens the risk of abnormalities in breast tissue.

To supplement with iodine, we take a drop of Lugol's 5 percent iodine in a large glass of water every four or five days. Iodine is best taken with magnesium because the body needs it to use iodine. Food sources for iodine are seafood, including sea vegetables, and dark-green leafy vegetables. This means that iodine isn't a big part of the American diet. The little seaweed that Americans eat is usually nori in sushi, and among the types of seaweed, nori is one of the lowest in iodine. Seaweed salad made of kombu, kelp, wakame, dulse, or hijiki contains much more iodine than nori does. Seafood in general is also high in iodine, so the safe fishes we listed in chapters 4 and 5 help with iodine level.

Working with a holistic physician to test iodine and thyroid hormone levels is the best way to see if you're getting enough iodine. You can also do a quick test to get a feel for your iodine level: put a drop of Lugol's 5 percent iodine on your forearm. The drop should leave a dark-orange stain on the skin that slowly fades as the iodine is absorbed through your skin into your body. If the stain is gone within four hours, there's a good chance you're deficient in iodine, but if it's still there after twenty-four hours, your body probably has plenty of iodine. You've just witnessed your body's amazing ability to absorb substances it needs through the skin and repel substances it doesn't need.

Remember to be careful when you're correcting an iodine deficiency—too much iodine is very dangerous. If you get a runny nose after taking a drop or two of Lugol's iodine in water, you've probably had a bit too much and would do well to back off for a few days. But that doesn't mean your iodine level is sufficient yet. It just means you had a bit too much at once.

Probiotics

Probiotics are one of the best supplements you can take to avoid an intestinal imbalance. They strengthen the intestinal walls and manufacture vital nutrients. They also help the body to use nutrients and fight harmful microbes in the GI tract. Your body actually contains about ten times as many probiotic bacteria cells as it does human cells! You simply couldn't survive without these little creatures. Probiotics protect us from a number of health problems, including food allergies and skin problems.

Probiotics also play a key role in the female reproductive system. Like the GI tract, the vagina contains and relies on a delicate ecosystem for optimal health. The *Lactobacillus* strains that populate the walls of the vagina make the environment too acidic for most intruders, thus protecting the vagina and the womb from infection. Just like the GI tract, however, this ecosystem can easily become disrupted by the exact same causes: antibiotics and stress. Spermicides and birth control pills can also cause an imbalance. Imbalances can usually be remedied with therapeutic doses of *Lactobacillus acidophilus*.

When you buy probiotic supplements, it's important to know which strains of probiotic bacteria are in the supplement. Each strain and substrain offers its own unique benefits. The *Lactobacillus* and *Bifidobacterium* strains are found naturally in the human GI tract and offer countless health benefits. They're the most prevalent strains you'll find in supplements. *Lactobacillus GG*, sold as Culturelle, is the best studied.

Bacillus subtilis is a wonderfully beneficial probiotic that does not occur naturally in humans but is found in many probiotic supplements. It's excellent at killing pathogens and unwanted microorganisms. If *B. subtilis* is on the ingredients list of your probiotic supplement, you have a gentle friend offering powerful protection.

Probiotic supplements come in capsules and powders. They're alive yet dormant when you get them in this form and become active when exposed to warmth and moisture inside your body. Either form is fine, but it's critical to take them on an empty stomach (when your stomach acid levels are low). Even though they can live in the intestines, most probiotics don't survive stomach acid. Enteric-coated capsules help, too.

During pregnancy, the advantage to taking probiotic supplements instead of fermented probiotic sources like kombucha, kefir, or yogurt is that the exact strains you're getting are tightly controlled. The cultures used in fermented foods aren't always tightly controlled, so you run the risk of ingesting organisms like yeasts, which produce toxins.

Krill or Fish Oil

Fish oil and krill oil (but not cod liver oil) are high in omega-3 fatty acids, an essential component of any healthy diet. Omega-3 lowers harmful cholesterol levels and has displayed a number of other cardiovascular benefits, including improved blood viscosity and fat levels. Studies have shown that people who eat more omega-3 fatty acids have lower rates of heart attack than people who eat less. The omega-3 fatty acids in fish oil also reduce the symptoms of inflammatory and immune disorders like Crohn's disease, ulcerative colitis, psoriasis, multiple sclerosis, and migraine headaches.

One of the omega-3 fatty acids, docosahexaenoic acid (DHA), plays a central role in the function of synaptic connections (communication points) in the brain. Because of this, the brain and the nerves are so dependent on DHA for proper function that a diet chronically deficient in DHA can result in degeneration of the nervous system. For example, a low DHA level has been associated with a higher rate of multiple sclerosis, schizophrenia, depression, dementia, and Alzheimer's disease. Omega-3 sufficiency has been associated with improved brain performance.

Omega-3, especially DHA, plays a key role in fetal brain development. High omega-3 intake during the third trimester boosts sensory, cognitive, and motor development in infants. The brain greatly increases in size during the last trimester, and it needs a lot of omega-3 to do it correctly. New mothers have been found to have half the omega-3 blood level of a man or of a woman who isn't pregnant or lactating. That's how much omega-3 fatty acids a baby needs to develop. So much of a mother's omega-3 is fed to the baby that if she doesn't replace it, she'll barely have any left for herself or for her future babies. This has been suggested as a cause of firstborn children scoring higher on intelligence tests.

A sufficient amount of omega-3 will also optimize vision in infants and prevent premature delivery. This makes fish oil or krill oil one of the most important supplements a woman can take during pregnancy, especially for having a smarter baby. Fish oil is also an important supplement for aspiring fathers, because DHA is required to make healthy sperm.

Breast milk, which is naturally high in DHA, is even higher in it if the mother consumes extra omega-3. Breast-fed babies have been shown to be more intelligent than formula-fed babies. A 2002 study suggests that these intelligence levels may stay with the babies into adulthood—so adults who were breast-fed as infants are smarter than their formula-fed peers. The difference is attributed to the high DHA content of breast milk boosting early brain development. Until very recently, formulas in the United States did not contain any DHA, and now only some do. Unfortunately, most pregnant women probably aren't eating enough omega-3 to support their baby's brain development properly.

Another omega-3 fatty acid, alpha-linolenic acid (ALA), is found in plant oils like flax and hemp. We prefer fish or krill oil for good reason: the DHA and the eicosapentaenoic acid (EPA) in fish and krill oil are more biologically potent than the ALA is, and even though our bodies can make DHA and EPA from ALA, it's not done very efficiently. It is estimated that only 1 to 4 percent of consumed ALA will typically be converted to DHA. The rest creates an overload of ALA.

We recommend supplementing with fish or krill oil but not cod liver oil. It's our opinion that most cod liver oil, or liver oil in general, will contain too much fully formed vitamin A to be consumed during pregnancy. Too much vitamin A is harmful because it blocks vitamin D from working, as we noted earlier.

Krill oil is more expensive than fish oil, but if you have room in your budget, it's the better choice of the two; that's because the omega-3 in krill oil is more easily used by the body and is less susceptible to oxidation. The DHA and EPA in krill oil are in the form of phospholipids, whereas the DHA and EPA in fish oil are usually triglycerides. Since phospholipids are the building blocks of our cell membranes, krill omega-3 packaged in phospholipids is more easily absorbed into the cells for use.

Also, since DHA and EPA are very polyunsaturated, they're fragile and oxidize easily—so easily, in fact, that many fish oil supplements are oxidized during the manufacturing process or from exposure to sunlight. Oxidized supplements are not only less helpful, they're harmful, because they burden the body. The phospholipids in krill oil aren't as susceptible to oxidation, so the chances you're getting high-quality, beneficial DHA and EPA are much higher if you choose krill.

Brain Nutrients

There are a handful of nutrients that promote brain development and function in adults and babies. We'll go through each one separately, but many supplement manufacturers bundle them together in a single brain formula. Check our website, www.betterbabybook.com/brain, for details on the best formulas we've found.

Vitamins B5 and B12, which we've already discussed, are the most important vitamins for brain energy. They're central to brain development from the moment of conception,

Alpha GPC

Alpha GPC (the GPC stands for "glycerylphosphorylcholine") is a choline compound found naturally in the brain. It helps choline cross the blood-brain barrier, so it's an important component in supplying the brain (both yours and your baby's) with choline, which is critical for brain function and for fetal brain development. Alpha GPC is also a precursor to a critical brain neurotransmitter called acetylcholine. Choline is critical for brain function and for fetal brain development.

Alpha GPC works with growth-hormone releasing hormone to naturally stimulate the production of human growth hormone. And by boosting choline availability in the brain and throughout the body, alpha GPC promotes liver health by reducing fatty liver conditions, which are associated with liver failure.

Most alpha GPC is made from highly purified soy lecithin. It's taken as a dietary supplement to enhance memory and brain power. A 1994 Italian study found that alpha GPC assisted the cognitive recovery of patients who had suffered a recent stroke.

Do not supplement with alpha GPC if you have excessive muscle or jaw tension; it could make it worse.

Glutamine

Glutamine is the most abundant amino acid in the human body and is a key component in muscle structure and nerve function. Amino acids make up proteins, which are the primary construction elements in your body. The body can make glutamine on its own, so technically it's a nonessential amino acid. Practically speaking, though, the body could not go on without glutamine. In times of high physical activity like pregnancy, the body often doesn't make enough glutamine to keep up with demand, so the answer is to take extra. More than 60 percent of muscle mass is glutamine. The body can convert glutamine to glucose and use it as an energy source.

Glutamine can easily cross the blood-brain barrier. Inside the brain, glutamine is transformed into glutamic acid and GABA, one of the chief neurotransmitters of the central nervous system. During normal brain function, amino acids change chemically inside the brain. This causes the release of individual ammonia structures. Too much loose ammonia in the brain becomes toxic and impairs brain and nerve function. Glutamic acid binds with these free ammonia structures and carries them out of the brain.

Since glutamine is so important to the nervous system, the body will pull it from the muscles during times of stress to keep the nervous system running, leading to muscle deterioration and loss. Muscle breakdown due to stress is therefore greatly curbed if you supplement with glutamine during a stressful time. Because of its important role in the nervous system, glutamine is a mandatory brain food. Glutamine sufficiency supports long-term optimal mental performance.

We recommend supplementing with glutamine during pregnancy because it contributes so much to body construction and nerve function. Your baby's muscular and neural development depends heavily on the presence of glutamine. Pregnancy is also stressful sometimes, and delivery, of course, is highly stressful. Proper glutamine intake is essential to maintaining muscular integrity and brain function in mother and baby during this time.

Acetyl-L-Carnitine

Acetyl-L-carnitine (ALC) is a nutrient that carries raw energy sources like carbohydrates and fatty acids from outside the cells into the mitochondria, which are the power plants inside the cells. Mitochondria take the raw resources and turn them into adenosine triphosphate (ATP) through the Krebs cycle (the citric acid cycle). ATP is the primary fuel that cells use to function. Every cell in your body contains mitochondria, and some cells, like heart cells, have far more mitochondria than other cells.

Mitochondria function throughout the body declines with age. This decline can be caused by a diet that is deficient in some of the nutrients required for the Krebs cycle to complete properly. It can also be caused by free radical damage, to which mitochondria are very susceptible.

Making sure that your diet contains all of the nutrients for the Krebs cycle will help to maintain optimal mitochondria function. This is where ALC comes in.

ALC plays a key role in keeping cells functioning, because without it they would run out of raw resources, even if there were plenty of these resources located right outside the cell. The cell would then run out of fuel, shut down, and die. This would be similar to running out of gas while driving, having extra gas to put in the car in a separate container, but having no way to get the extra gas into the car's gas tank. If cells run out of raw energy sources on a large scale, the person loses energy, vitality, and eventually his or her life. Long-chain fatty acids, which are one of the most concentrated sources of energy, have a particularly difficult time entering cells without ALC. Finally, the acetyl group that is part of ALC is central to the production of the neurotransmitter acetylcholine in the brain.

Supplementing with ALC improves mitochondria function, which improves energy level, brain function, and memory and is an important ingredient in fetal brain development. ALC is a natural overall performance enhancer. While plain L-carnitine will help with energy production, the brain development and performance benefits are mostly to be had only from ALC. This is true because ALC crosses the blood-brain barrier much more easily than L-carnitine does.

The higher energy production and mental clarity from ALC naturally causes other processes to run more effectively and smoothly throughout the body. Simultaneously, ALC protects us from certain disorders and ailments. Many people who supplement with ALC have said that it makes them feel more mentally focused and alert. Taking it regularly can lead to improved memory, help to restore basic mental function in a senile brain, slow the progression of Alzheimer's disease, and help with ADHD in children with fragile X syndrome, an X chromosome–linked inherited disorder. ALC also reduces fatigue and increases male sexual function and sperm motility. All of these benefits come with no observed side effects.

The most important reasons to take ALC during pregnancy are its ability to cross the blood-brain barrier and the central role it plays in the production of acetylcholine in the brain, which is crucial for fetal brain development.

Phosphatidylserine

Phosphatidylserine (PS) is found in cell walls throughout the body, and it helps nutrients to enter the cells and waste products to leave them. Supplementing with PS can support memory and cognition, reduce exercise-related stress, prevent physiological deterioration in athletes, and enhance mood during mental stress. There isn't any research on taking PS during pregnancy, but because foods are typically low in PS, we did supplement with it during pregnancy by using organic soy lecithin, which contains 10 to 20 milligrams of PS per hundred grams. PS supplements are usually expensive, so using non-GMO soy lecithin is a cheap way to get plenty of extra PS. Sunflower lecithin is an even better way to get PS because of concerns about estrogenic soy compounds escaping into soy lecithin. We used soy lecithin for both our children but would have used sunflower lecithin if it was available then.

Brain Nutrients to Avoid during Pregnancy

We suggest supplementing with the brain nutrients we just mentioned separately or finding a formula that does *not* contain any of the following: ginkgo biloba, vinpocetine, huperzine A, and dimethylethanolamine (DMAE).

Ginkgo biloba is an herb that increases blood flow to the brain. There's evidence that it may help with intermittent claudication (leg weakness and cramping caused by poor circulation), dementia, cerebrovascular insufficiency (inadequate blood flow in the brain), macular degeneration, and tinnitus. It also helps to mitigate altitude sickness, vertigo, premenstrual syndrome, and age-related memory loss.

The main concern with using ginkgo during pregnancy is its anti-platelet activity. Theoretically, this could prolong bleeding during delivery. Considering this, we didn't think ginkgo was a necessary addition to our plan. If you choose to use ginkgo during pregnancy, we recommend discontinuing use in the last trimester. Also, if you take ginkgo, make sure you get it from a good manufacturing practices facility—toxins have been found in poorly produced ginkgo supplements.

Like ginkgo, vinpocetine enhances blood flow to the brain, and it also protects neurons. It's a synthetically altered form of vincamine, an extract from the periwinkle plant. Vinpocetine is used primarily as a vasodilator (to widen the blood vessels) and a memory enhancer.

Huperzine A is a naturally occurring compound found in the firmoss plant. It enhances memory and has been used in the treatment of Alzheimer's disease. Since vinpocetine and huperzine A aren't brain-building blocks and their use during pregnancy hasn't been well studied, we chose to avoid them during pregnancy.

DMAE increases the brain's choline level. It's been shown to increase vigilance, alertness, and attention span and promote a positive mood. Research suggests that it may help children with ADHD. DMAE is contraindicated during pregnancy because it's been found to cause growth retardation in developing mouse embryos, including neural tube defects. There are other, safer ways of increasing brain choline concentration during pregnancy, like taking alpha GPC or simply eating choline in raw egg yolks and lecithin.

Antioxidants

An antioxidant inhibits oxidation, the reaction promoted by free radicals that we discussed in chapter 4. When you supply your body with enough of the right antioxidants, you will be able to protect your cells—and your baby—from free radicals that can harm cells. Many antioxidants are also potent detoxifyers.

Coenzyme Q10

Coenzyme Q10 (coQ10) is an antioxidant that helps the body to neutralize free radicals. It's also a key part of mitochondrial respiration and helps the body to produce ATP, the primary fuel of cells. CoQ10 is able to reactivate used vitamins C and E throughout the body.

As an antioxidant, coQ10 increases fertility, especially in men. Taking it helps with pregnancy, because the placenta contains a lot of it. CoQ10 in the placenta protects the baby from oxidation and helps to prevent preeclampsia. This is a big factor in preventing birth defects, because preeclampsia can lead to malnutrition and the subsequent slow growth of the fetus. A low coQ10 level is correlated with spontaneous abortion. It's important to take coQ10 during lactation, too. Breast milk functions as an antioxidant, and coQ10 is largely responsible for that. When a mother supplements with coQ10, her breast milk will contain plenty to protect her baby.

CoQ10 supplements usually come oxidized, which means that the body needs to activate them before they can do their job. If a coQ10 supplement is bright orange in color, it's already oxidized. If you're under age thirty, normal oxidized coQ10 works just fine and is affordable. After age thirty, the body has a hard time activating CoQ10. If you're over thirty, we recommend using a reduced (preactivated) coQ10 supplement called ubiquinol. This is usually more expensive.

If you've ever taken statin drugs for cholesterol, we believe it's imperative to supplement with coQ10 from preconception through lactation. It's well documented that statin drugs quickly use up the body's coQ10 supply.

Liposomal Glutathione

Glutathione is one of the most powerful antioxidants. It's a tripeptide (a group of three amino acids) formed from L-cystine, L-glutamic acid, and glycine. The liver uses glutathione to deal with toxins all the time. Glutathione protects cells from free radicals and other cell-damaging reactive molecules, including those found in acrylonitrile, a common plasticizer and auto exhaust toxin found in the air. It also helps to detoxify air pollution, alcohol, antipsychotic and antiepileptic drugs, cigarette smoke, heavy metals, hyperoxia (excess oxygen in the blood), mycotoxins, pesticides, radiation, thalidomide, and the estrogenic chemical vinyl chloride found in a wide variety of PVC plastics. Like coQ10, glutathione reactivates used vitamins C and E.

Glutathione is a powerful force in maintaining a mother's body as an ideal, safe environment for her fetus. Like coQ10, glutathione is highly concentrated in the placenta, so taking plenty before conception and during the first trimester could help to prevent birth defects. In the placenta, glutathione neutralizes toxins and pollutants before they ever reach the fetus. It also increases fertility, especially in men.

We each took a teaspoon of liposomal (fat-encapsulated) glutathione every day for six months before Lana got pregnant. When you supplement with glutathione, it's important to buy liposomal glutathione. It is manufactured in such a way that the glutathione molecules are wrapped in healthy fats. These fats escort the glutathione right into the cells, making it far more useful to the body than nonliposomal glutathione supplements. In cell culture studies, liposomal glutathione has been shown to be a hundred times more effective than regular reduced glutathione.

You can also raise the glutathione level in the body by taking glutathione precursors. Two of these, N-acetyl-cysteine and selenium, were recently shown to improve fertility in men. We did everything we could to make sure that Dave's sperm had normal structure and form, so he took the precursors as well as fully formed liposomal glutathione. The most effective brands are at www.betterbabybook.com/antioxidants.

8

Hormones and Pharmaceuticals

Thanks to cutting-edge science, there are a few things you can do to enhance your unborn baby's growth and development that go beyond epigenetics. This chapter is about supplementing with the hormone progesterone and potential improvements in baby health and intelligence that could come from two pharmaceutical drugs.

The idea of using pharmaceuticals to create healthier babies is controversial. There are huge ethical questions. Will we grow into a society where everyone has to take pharmaceuticals to have kids who can "keep up"? Should we use pharmaceuticals that increase intelligence but cause a small increase in birth defects?

We're uncomfortable with these questions, but we also believe that this book wouldn't be complete without touching on the most promising substances with near zero risk. You should not use any pharmaceutical during pregnancy without your doctor's help. This is not an area for self-experimentation.

Since Lana is a doctor and we both know a great deal about how bodies work, we knew that using some of these substances would be safe even if they didn't enhance the health of our children. The benefits of progesterone on Lana were quite obvious (no morning sickness, vibrant skin, stable moods). Based on the research in this chapter, we believe it probably also helped our children to maximize their potential. In any case, we don't suggest experimenting on your own without first consulting a holistic doctor.

Progesterone

We can thank Katharina Dalton, a London-based physician who defined the term PMS in the 1950s, for the first research on the effects of progesterone use during pregnancy. In the 1960s, she found that children born to mothers who used progesterone were more advanced in development at one year old and performed better academically at ages nine and ten than their peers did. Dalton reported that children whose mothers received more than five grams of prenatal progesterone performed best academically and were more likely to go to college. These "progesterone babies," as she called them, became famous after her study. Although she didn't believe progesterone would produce a race of geniuses, she thought it would ensure full brain development.

Dalton's methods were later questioned in 1978 when studies led by Anthony Lynch at the Department of Psychology, University of Keele, in Staffordshire England, contradicted her conclusion. In addition, a 2006 study concluded that not enough is known about progesterone to be sure it's safe to use during pregnancy. We took this into consideration, but after talking with other antiaging and endocrine experts, we decided that using an appropriate amount of bioidentical progesterone during pregnancy to offset the artificially high estrogen in our environment would produce positive results.

Progesterone facilitates optimal brain development. It helps to prevent preterm delivery, which promotes more complete fetal development. It protects the neurons of a fetus by suppressing the excitation that is capable of damaging fragile new brain tissue. Progesterone has also been shown to heal injured brain tissue in adults. It decreases stress and increases a feeling of well-being in the mother, producing calmer babies. From the perspective of epigenetics, a lower stress level in the mother would certainly help to sustain growth programs in her baby. We don't know whether progesterone leads to an increase in intelligence, but we were happy to enjoy the protective benefits.

We also believe that progesterone use can prevent stretch marks, since too little progesterone and too much estrogen contribute to their formation. Although this isn't proven, Lana didn't develop any stretch marks through two pregnancies while using progesterone. Vitamin C may have played a role there, too.

Beware of Synthetic Progesterone

In any kind of hormone replacement therapy, it's very important to use bioidentical products. *Bioidentical* means that a substance, though created in a lab, is identical to the substance found in nature. Bioidentical progesterone is the exact same type of progesterone that's found in your body, and it's the only progesterone that works. At the time that Dalton did her studies in the late 1960s, bioidentical progesterone was used.

What other progesterone exists? Since pharmaceutical companies cannot legally patent progesterone itself, they tweak the molecule a bit and then market it as an effective progesterone supplement that they can sell for expensive prices. Many doctors do not understand the difference between these impostor drugs and real progesterone, so it's critical to make sure you know this information.

Depo-Provera is a synthetic form of progesterone that has a different effect inside the body. It's largely similar to bioidentical progesterone, but it is slightly altered (presumably so it could be patented). Depo-Provera is so damaging to the female reproductive system that it's used as a form of birth control. It interferes with hormone signaling to prevent eggs from being released from the ovaries. This happens because Depo-Provera binds more strongly to the part of cells where progesterone binds than natural progesterone does, while not conferring the same benefits on mother and baby that real progesterone does. David Zava, a biochemist at ZRT Laboratory in Beaverton, Oregon, explains that progesterone is a "master key" that unlocks a number of bodily functions. Although Depo-Provera does shut down the ovaries effectively, it doesn't calm the nervous system or stabilize the cardiovascular system as bioidentical progesterone does. Depo-Provera is also rife with harmful side effects, because it blocks a woman's body from using its own natural supply of progesterone. Using bioidentical progesterone certainly won't prevent pregnancy, as Depo-Provera does.

In *What Your Doctor May Not Tell You about Menopause: The Breakthrough Book on Natural Hormone Balance*, Dr. John Lee points out that Depo-Provera causes a "terrible incidence of side effects." Women often feel terrible when using it. The 1993 *Physician's Desk Reference* states that Depo-Provera can contribute to heart and limb defects in a fetus if it is used during the first four months of pregnancy. The use of synthetic progesterone during pregnancy has also been shown to measurably alter personality in the fetus and restrict circulation. Depo-Provera is a hormone disrupter that's about as dangerous as the mycotoxins we describe elsewhere in this book. Don't ever use it, and always be wary of hormone replacements that aren't bioidentical.

Getting Started with Progesterone

If you choose to use bioidentical progesterone during pregnancy, we recommend getting a full hormone analysis first and working with a holistic antiaging doctor to optimize your levels. For any hormone, getting the dosage correct is critical—if you don't, adverse side effects can result.

Hormones usually aren't taken orally because the liver and digestive system will filter most of them out for excretion. Using a cream that soaks into the skin is an effective way to bypass the liver and get progesterone into the body, but the cream often results in a high progesterone level. This is because over time the progesterone is stored in high quantities in fatty skin tissue instead of being used or excreted. We've found that the best way to use progesterone is in the form that dissolves under the tongue and flows directly into the bloodstream. It's much more difficult to overdose with the sublingual form, and it doesn't build up in your body the way the cream can.

Deprenyl

Deprenyl is a pharmaceutical substance that has been proven to reduce the age-related decline of the neurotransmitter dopamine. It increases dopamine availability throughout the brain, thereby preserving youthful brain function. Dopamine plays a key role in a variety of brain functions, including behavior, cognition, voluntary movement, motivation, fear, sleep, mood, attention, working memory, and learning. It's usually associated with the brain's reward system, so it also plays a key role in a person's experience of happiness. Besides increasing dopamine, Deprenyl has been found to promote optimal levels of other key neurotransmitters, like serotonin, norepinephrine, and epinephrine.

Deprenyl was originally developed as a mental energizer with antidepressant effects. It may even be able to extend the life span by slowing the death rate of nigral neurons, a tiny group of nerves that are essential for dopamine synthesis and function. After about age forty-five, the nigral neurons die off at a rate of about 13 percent per decade, reducing a person's vigor, life force, and the intensity of their life experience. This means that even if a person reached age 115 in perfect health, they're still likely to die due to a shortage of nigral neurons. Studies on rats and dogs have shown Deprenyl to be a powerful life-extension agent. In the United States, Deprenyl is now used in the treatment of Parkinson's disease. It's also been shown to increase sexual function and desire and to help with senile dementia, learning disorders, and a host of other ailments. In other words, when used at lower antiaging doses, Deprenyl is an amazing drug.

There is a case for using very small doses of Deprenyl during pregnancy for several reasons. It's been shown to protect nerve cells from a number of neurotoxins by strengthening neuronal membranes. It's safe— in a 2008 study on the effects of Deprenyl during pregnancy, it was found to have no detrimental effects on rat embryo development, even when used in doses much higher than those prescribed for humans. Not only did Deprenyl cause no harm, the study concluded that overall Deprenyl actually enhanced embryonic quality. It may even improve intelligence, by stimulating more neural connections. We've experienced sharper brain function ourselves while using Deprenyl.

Deprenyl comes in several forms and is sold under a few different names. There are patches, tablets, and a liquid. We recommend the liquid, which is called liquid Deprenyl citrate (LDC). LDC is the purest form of Deprenyl available. Deprenyl is sold as Selegiline, Jumex, Selepryl, Eldepryl, and Cyprenil. For the neuroprotective and neuroenhancing qualities, a *very* low dose of two milligrams per day is enough, and only during the second and third trimester. That is approximately 5 percent of the normal pharmaceutical dosage.

When Deprenyl is taken in such small doses well into pregnancy, though, we believe that the neuroprotective benefits outweigh whatever risks there may be.

Before using a pharmaceutical drug like Deprenyl during pregnancy, you must consult with an antiaging or holistic physician familiar with very small doses of Deprenyl. Deprenyl is a prescription drug, so you'll need to work with a physician who's willing to prescribe it for use during pregnancy. Pregnancy is not an accepted use for Deprenyl, despite this research, so you may not be able to find a physician willing to prescribe it. For the health of our children, this is something in our medical system that ought to change. We would have liked to have had a prescription for Deprenyl for use during both pregnancies.

Oxiracetam

Oxiracetam is a nontoxic, water-soluble drug that has been proven to increase brain performance. It was originally developed by the Italian pharmaceutical company ICF. A member of the racetam family of brain-enhancing drugs, oxiracetam is a more potent, more effective version of piracetam, the original racetam.

Oxiracetam has demonstrated lots of benefits while showing no detectable adverse side effects, even when taken in very large doses. Although it does not affect cerebral blood flow, it increases brain concentrations of the cellular energy source adenosine triphosphate. Scores of studies have demonstrated that oxiracetam increases brainpower. A 1986 study showed that oxiracetam enhanced vigilance in elderly people with dementia.

In 1988, Italian researchers tested oxiracetam on pregnant mice to see if it caused birth defects. No birth defects whatsoever were observed, and the one-month-old pups of the mother mice given oxi-racetam were more curious than their peers. At three months old, the pups demonstrated significantly better performance on memory tests. A 1989 study of 272 people with dementia showed that oxiracetam improved their concentration and memory. In animal testing, oxirace-tam has been shown to reduce the negative effects of harmful exposure to microwaves.

We used oxiracetam during pregnancy for two reasons. First, it pro-tects brain cells in the event of low oxygen, which lowers the risk of oxygen-related brain damage in the womb. Second, we were familiar with its benefits and wanted to pass along the benefits of higher brain ATP to our children. Oxiracetam has been proven to be exceptionally safe even in large doses. Although we can't quantify the benefits, we are certain that oxiracetam was safer to take than even Tylenol.

There are stronger racetam drugs available, like aniracetam, but these are usually oil-soluble. We therefore don't recommend using them—or other oil-soluble pharmaceuticals—during pregnancy for the reason of potential toxicity. If the body needs to eliminate a substance, water-soluble substances are far easier to eliminate than oil-soluble substances.

Oxiracetam has been sold in Italy since 1988. It can be found under the names CT-848, hydroxy-piracetam, ISF-2522, Neuractiv, and Neuromet. In the United States, oxiracetam is pending FDA approval for use in treating Alzheimer's disease. You'll probably need to work with a doctor to get oxiracetam.

A Warning about Pharmaceuticals

We chose to use some of these pharmaceutical drugs because we very much understood what they could do for our babies and our own bodies at the molecular level. We exhaustively researched the risks until we were certain they were near zero, and we were very conservative with our dose. As a physician, Lana was able to determine the appropriate dos-ages. Even then, we got second opinions from other experts. We believe that these pharmaceutical drugs are safe and effective and actually lower pregnancy risk.

With our current legal system, no pharmaceutical company will ever market a drug that makes for healthier, smarter babies. The liability is too high no matter how compelling the research may be. We hope that by discussing these pharmaceuticals here, we can bring to light some of the potential for health and wellness in our children.

Please do not take this as encouragement to experiment with pharmaceuticals while pregnant. The results could be disastrous for you and your children. Work with physicians and always choose near-zero-risk options that offer more benefits than risk. It's not worth risking birth defects—or even death—to have a healthier baby.

PART THREE

The Toxin Connection

9

How Mold Changes Your Pregnancy

Toxins cause health problems for everyone, but the problems are less severe for an adult than for a fetus. Adults have fully formed blood-brain barriers and mature immune systems. In the womb, a fetus is somewhat protected from toxins by the mother's ability to filter them, but some toxins get through, and babies aren't prepared to deal with them the way adults are.

There are so many toxins and pollutants that it's not useful to list each one—there are thousands. It's easier to understand the main categories of toxins, where they come from, what they do, and what you can do to keep them from affecting your pregnancy.

Toxins come from three main sources: your food, your environment, and inside your body. A shocking number of common ailments—some life-threatening—are the result of chronic exposure to low levels of toxins. Most people don't know this because they don't feel the effects soon enough to realize that the toxins are the cause of their health problems.

Just like slowly dripping water can erode limestone, low levels of toxins erode health over time.

Toxins erode a fetus's health and neurological development much more quickly, however. Imagine water dripping slowly on soft soil instead of limestone. A fetus is more sensitive because it's growing so quickly. If a fetus is exposed to toxins that distort DNA—and many toxins do—the altered DNA is translated to all future cells that grow from the damaged cell. In an adult body, a poisoned cell is just one of billions of cells. An adult is able to flush that cell out of the body and continue normal operation. This is why it takes much more of a toxin to harm an adult than it does a fetus.

For an embryo or a fetus, the damaged cell is responsible for being the parent of billions of cells. If toxins have distorted the parent cell's DNA, all the billions of cells it produces through mitosis (cell division) can be distorted as well. This is why birth defects are so prevalent and why an unborn baby is much more susceptible to damage from toxins than an adult is. If the tiniest toxin comes into contact with the wrong cell during rapid fetal growth, the entire growth pattern can be derailed. This is why our plan protects your baby from as many toxins as possible.

Toxins in Food

There is a blurry line between foods that are simply bad for us and foods that are toxic. For instance, even a little too much sugar is bad for you because it causes harmful processes in the body, but sugar is not toxic. In contrast, fish is now often contaminated with mercury, and mercury is highly toxic. Fried foods are both bad for us and toxic. They contain oxidized oils that are stressful for the body to handle (bad for you), but the high temperatures used in frying overheat the starchy breading and create carcinogenic toxins called tricyclic amines.

Common toxins in food include artificial additives, preservatives, and colorings. In chapter 4, we explained which foods should be avoided because of toxins.

Mycotoxins are the most insidious and little-known food toxins. Fungi, like molds and yeasts, produce them for protection. Mycotoxins are common in crops because trace amounts of mold grew on the food and secreted mycotoxins long before the food was harvested. Governments often limit the concentration of a few mycotoxins in the food supply, but the limits aren't strict enough for optimal health. Some types of mycotoxins aren't regulated at all. Even though mycotoxins aren't commonly talked about, avoiding them is central to a healthy pregnancy.

Mycotoxins are extremely small molecules that are undetectable by the human immune system. This is what makes them so sinister—the body doesn't see them, so it doesn't fight them or eliminate them effectively. Mycotoxins are harmful to people in extremely small concentrations, measured in parts per billion. Because they're so small, they cross the placenta and reach your baby easily.

Poisoning from mycotoxins can be difficult to detect. Some mycotoxins produce symptoms right away, but others produce no symptoms until the condition is quite advanced. Exposure to mycotoxins over time can cause infertility and a number of pregnancy-related problems, including spontaneous abortion. Mycotoxins also contribute to cancer and even autism.

Grains are the most commonly contaminated foods. A recent study in Asia and Europe found that 58 percent of animal feed samples were contaminated. Sometimes dangerous levels are found in our food supply as well. Animal products like meat and milk can be contaminated because the animals are fed grains. These animal products often pose a higher mycotoxin risk than the grains we eat, because the mycotoxin controls on animal feed are much more lenient than the controls on the grains in our food supply. Mycotoxins are one of the reasons we recommend eating only products from 100 percent grass-fed or pastured animals. Pasture grasses are very low in mycotoxins.

Types of Mycotoxins

The major types of mycotoxins are aflatoxin, ergot alkaloids, fumonisin, trichothecenes, ochratoxin, and zearalenone. Each type occurs in certain climates and is prone to contaminating certain crops. To keep mycotoxins away from your baby, you should become familiar with the different types.

Aflatoxin

Found on: Corn, cottonseed, and peanuts.

Produced by: *Aspergillus* molds in hot, dry weather. Aflatoxin is one of the most toxic substances on Earth. Even trace amounts are harmful, especially for a baby.

Ergot alkaloids

Found on: Rye, triticale, barley, wheat, and oats.

Produced by: Ergot molds in cool, wet weather. It infects grain heads, replacing healthy kernels with dark formations called sclerotia. Ergot has been linked to infertility in farm animals and changes in nervous systems and blood flow.

Fumonisin

Found on: Corn. Fresh sweet corn (organic) is usually okay; dried corn is usually contaminated.

Produced by: Fusarium molds worldwide. Fumonisin disrupts the growth of cell membranes. For a fast-growing fetus, toxins like fumonisin are especially difficult to handle.

Trichothecenes

Found on: Corn, wheat, soybeans, and cereal grains.

Produced by: Fusarium and related red and purple molds worldwide. Trichothecenes are linked to greatly decreased fertility. One famous tricothecine is known as vomitoxin or deoxynivalenol. As the name implies, it causes extreme nausea and vomiting at very tiny doses. You don't want this when you're pregnant!

Ochratoxin

Found on: Barley, beer, cocoa, coffee, corn, many dried foods, fruit juices, legumes, malt, milk and cheese, nuts, oats, pork, poultry, rye, spices, wheat, and wine.

Produced by: *Aspergillus* and *Penicillium* molds in cool, wet conditions. Ochratoxins cause similar damage to health and fertility as other mycotoxins do. They're often found in the fat of animals that have consumed contaminated feed—that's why you'll find them in animal products. Ochratoxin levels are not controlled in the United States.

Zearalenone

Found on: Bananas, barley, corn, sorghum, and wheat.
Produced by: Fusarium molds in cool, wet weather. If corn is heavily infected, it may have a dark-purple discoloration, and if wheat is infected, it is typical to see pink tips. Zearalenone is a powerful estrogen hormone disrupter and has been linked to more damaging effects than any other mycotoxin.

Locations of Mycotoxins

Mycotoxins are more prevalent in some parts of the world than others. The following list shows the percentage of animal feed samples contaminated, by region:

North America

Aflatoxin: 16%
Fumonisin: 64%
Ochratoxin: 50%
Trichothecene (Deoxynivalenol): 68%
Zearalenone: 38%

South America

Aflatoxin: 59%
Fumonisin: 88%
Ochratoxin: 0%
Trichothecene (Deoxynivalenol): 24%
Zearalenone: 96%

Northern Europe

Aflatoxin: 0%
Fumonisin: 0%
Ochratoxin: 50%
Trichothecene (Deoxynivalenol): 50%
Zearalenone: 0%

Central Europe

Aflatoxin: 3%
Fumonisin: 22%
Ochratoxin: 45%
Trichothecene (Deoxynivalenol): 50%
Zearalenone: 15%

Southern Europe

Aflatoxin: 11%
Fumonisin: 25%
Ochratoxin: 25%
Trichothecene (Deoxynivalenol): 59%
Zearalenone: 13%

Middle East

Aflatoxin: 50%
Fumonisin: 11%
Ochratoxin: 67%
Trichothecene (Deoxynivalenol): 43%
Zearalenone: 0%

Africa

Aflatoxin: 72%
Fumonisin: 82%
Ochratoxin: 50%
Trichothecene (Deoxynivalenol): 50%
Zearalenone: 35%

North Asia

Aflatoxin: 10%
Fumonisin: 53%

Ochratoxin: 22%
Trichothecene (Deoxynivalenol): 83%
Zearalenone: 65%

South Asia

Aflatoxin: 79%
Fumonisin: 62%
Ochratoxin: 68%
Trichothecene (Deoxynivalenol): 15%
Zearalenone: 21%

Southeast Asia

Aflatoxin: 65%
Fumonisin: 61%
Ochratoxin: 34%
Trichothecene (Deoxynivalenol): 17%
Zearalenone: 50%

Australia

Aflatoxin: 17%
Fumonisin: 17%
Ochratoxin: 17%
Trichothecene (Deoxynivalenol): 17%
Zearalenone: 8%

Continental Europe and Australia pose the lowest overall risk, whereas South and Southeast Asia, South America, and Africa pose the largest threats. Note that the United States is widely exposed to mycotoxins. Different parts of the world are susceptible to different mycotoxins, so this list can help you find safe foods depending on where you are.

At the time of this writing, only three types of mycotoxins are regulated in the United States: aflatoxin, fumonisin, and trichothecenes. This means that the U.S. food supply is not rigorously tested for ochratoxin and zearalenone. Even though the United States has greater mycotoxin contamination than Europe, U.S. laws pay less heed to mycotoxins. While twenty parts per billion is standard for the human food supply in the United States, Europe has much tighter controls. Currently, Europe is striving for Codex Alimentarius (international food standards) import standards of only two parts per billion. We think the tighter controls in Europe are evidence that mycotoxins are a greater threat to health than many people realize.

Our bodies are so sensitive to mycotoxins that health problems result from concentrations lower than one hundred parts per billion. It rarely takes more, and it often takes much less. There's no known way to remove most mycotoxins from crops. Current controls can only prevent the molds from reaching the crops while they're growing, long before they reach feed mills or grocery stores.

Fortunately, there's a lot you can do to protect yourself from mycotoxins. Our diet (see chapters 4 and 5) is designed to help you avoid them. And when avoiding them isn't possible, you can use supplements like activated charcoal (see chapter 12), vitamin D3, and glutathione to remove them from the body.

10

Environmental Toxins

When most people think about environmental toxins these days, they think of the carbon dioxide level or oil spills. Although we're concerned about both of those for the good of the planet, they're unlikely to affect your unborn baby's cognitive development (unless you live near an oil spill). But there are many other types of environmental toxins that can affect a mother and fetus, even at low levels, including the following:

- Respiratory chain inhibitors: inhibit energy in cells
- Carcinogens: cause cancers
- Hormone disruptors: change sex characteristics in utero
- Neurotoxins: kill nerve cells
- Toxic metals (such as mercury, lead, arsenic, nickel, cadmium, and tin): linked to lower IQ and birth defects
- Environmental mycotoxins (such as airborne molds from water-damaged structures): have the same effects as other mycotoxins (see chapter 9)
- Electromagnetic fields: cause stress

In our daily lives, we're most commonly exposed to these environmental toxins through contact with these things:

- Petroleum products
- Plastics and the chemicals they contain
- Insecticides and household poisons, which can be hormone disruptors, neurotoxins, or respiratory chain inhibitors
- Household cleaning products, personal hygiene products, and cosmetics
- Flame retardants like PCBs
- Vehicle emissions near your home or office
- Volatile organic chemicals (VOCs), which are known to kill brain cells

In chapter 13 we'll deal with the toxins you're most likely to find in your home. Here we want to deal with the two most ubiquitous sources of environmental toxins: the air we breathe and the water we drink. Clean air and water are essential for a healthy pregnancy, but in many places, the air and water aren't so clean anymore. Industrialization creates an increasingly toxic environment around people in most countries. Here's a bit about our air and water and what you can do to keep them clean for your baby.

Air Pollutants

Breathing is the easiest way to be exposed to toxins. Factories, power plants, and automobiles constantly emit air contaminants like black carbon, particulate matter, and ozone. We usually don't notice, and we seem to go on living without any problems, but recent science has proven that air pollutants are present in concentrations that hurt us.

When a pregnant woman breathes polluted air, her baby is exposed to it as well. Today, women are exposed to polluted air like never before. Common air pollutants have been found throughout women's bodies, many of which pass through the placental barrier and threaten the baby. This happens in both urban and remote areas because Earth's air currents carry concentrated chemicals for thousands of miles. The pesticide DDT, used to control malaria in tropical regions, has been found high in the

Swiss Alps. Flame-retardant chemicals used in temperate climates have been found in the arctic circle. Many of these pollutants resemble the body's natural hormones. The body mistakes them, and communication in the body is disrupted. Disruption can occur in concentrations far below the regulated "safe" levels and can cause infertility.

Scientists haven't measured the extent of the damage these pollutants do, and there's not really a recipe for avoiding them completely. But there are steps we can take to keep the pollutants away from our unborn babies.

If you live in an urban area, you can take measures to purify the air in your home, or at least purify the air in your bedroom. The air inside your house is the air you breathe the most, and the air in your bedroom accounts for one-third of the air you breathe in your lifetime (assuming you're in bed eight hours a night). HEPA air purifiers are a great way to improve the air in your home—they remove 99.97 percent of airborne particles more than three-tenths of a micrometer in diameter.

If you live near a large metropolis like New York City or Los Angeles, it's a good idea to check the smog report before exercising outside. Weather reports in metropolitan areas typically issue ozone alerts and air-quality assessments each morning. If the air-quality reports are consistently bad where you live, consider doing less intense exercise outside and save intense exercise for a controlled environment with pure air. You can also avoid walking, running, or biking along streets with heavy traffic.

Water Pollutants

This is one of the most important things we say in this book: *drink only purified water.* These days, water from various sources is contaminated with harmful chemicals that industry releases into the environment. Some of these chemicals, like chlorine and fluorine, are even added on purpose. Here's a closer look at our water supply.

Tap Water

In a recent U.S. geological survey, traces of pharmaceutical drugs were found in the tap water of thirty states. The concentrations were bioactive—that is, still high enough to have an effect inside the body. It was reported that forty-one million Americans are exposed. Ninety-five different prescription and over-the-counter drugs were tested for, and painkillers, tranquilizers, antidepressants, antibiotics, birth control pills, and chemotherapy agents were found. Some of the water samples contained more than twenty drugs.

How do these drugs get into our water supply? The biggest contributor is likely to be livestock. More than 40 percent of all antibiotics are fed to cattle, whose manure is collected and used to fertilize farmland, gardens, and lawns. Once dispersed, the antibiotics are washed into the soil and into underground water sources. People also flush unused drugs down the toilet when they clean out their medicine cabinets, and hospitals do the same when disposing of old drugs. Used drugs are also naturally excreted as human waste into the sewer system.

All of these drugs end up in the sewer system, where they're routed to water treatment facilities. Most of these facilities are not capable of purifying water of drugs, so the drugs remain in the "clean" water that's routed back to homes and to your sink. The amount of drugs released into our environment every year is estimated to be more than eight hundred million pounds!

Drugs aren't the only toxins in our water supply. Heavy-metal by-products from industrial waste are common (such as mercury and nickel). Perchlorate (rocket fuel) has also been found. In 2008, the Environmental Protection Agency chose not to regulate rocket fuel content in the water supply, claiming that twenty-four and a half parts per billion are safe. Other research estimates that one part per billion should be the limit.

For our modern industrial environment, regulations on water purity are lax and outdated. In a December 2009 article, the *New York Times* acknowledged that significant quantities of more than sixty thousand toxic chemicals are used within the United States alone. Yet the thirty-five-year-old Safe Drinking Water Act regulates a mere ninety-one contaminants. Even worse, a December 2009 *New York Times* analysis of federal data concluded that in the last five years, more than 20 percent of U.S. water treatment systems have actually violated key provisions of the Safe Drinking Water Act, as lax as it may be.

Some toxic chemicals are intentionally added to our water. Chlorine is added as a disinfectant in municipalities throughout the United States. Many people think chlorine makes water safe. On the contrary, chlorine is as harmful to you as it is to the microbes in the water. In adults, chlorine injures the proteins that make up our bodies and promotes allergies and asthma. Pregnant women who drink water contaminated with chlorine by-products are at a higher risk of having babies with birth defects and central nervous system defects.

Fluorine (fluoride) is another highly toxic yet popular additive. We talk about fluorine in the section on toothpaste in chapter 13. Fluorine is added to water supplies in many (but not all) municipalities around the nation. Its use is based on the disproven theory that fluoride builds strong teeth.

The effects of chemicals in tap water are becoming evident. A 2006 study found that men who drank more than the commonly recommended eight (eight-ounce) glasses of tap water per day had a 50 percent higher risk of developing bladder cancer. The study found that this held true whether the water was consumed straight from the tap or boiled to make coffee or tea.

Well Water

Water from private wells should be tested at least once a year. All of the same contaminants that get into municipal water supplies aren't far from your well, and some of them, like industrial waste and pharmaceutical drugs, make their way directly into the underground water that supplies your well.

Filtered Water

In our experience, small sink attachments and water filter pitchers like Pur and Brita just aren't that thorough. Today's contaminants are often far too small (at the molecular level) for these filters to protect your unborn baby.

Bottled Water

Most bottled water comes in plastic bottles. Plastic often contains BPA, a harmful chemical that leaches into the water when the bottle is exposed to heat or sunlight. The chances are high that bottled water products have been exposed to heat or sunlight during shipping. Even if you find water bottled in glass, be sure to check the source or choose water tested for contaminants—some bottled water is actually just tap water! If you're sure of the source and quality, clean water bottled in glass is a smart choice.

The Solution

Unfortunately, the solution to getting clean water is a bit expensive. You'll need one of two things: a reverse-osmosis (RO) water purification system or a high-end countertop filtration unit. The contaminants we discussed above are often extremely small (even for molecules), and it takes a high-end system to remove them. RO and countertop filtration with carbon are the only systems robust enough to do the job.

If you're confident that you'll be living in your current residence for a long time, investing in an RO system is worth it. RO systems usually involve a professional, permanent installation that alters the plumbing around your kitchen sink. Countertop water filters are cheaper and more portable (you can take them with you when you move). They usually involve only a minimal alteration and connection to your tap. They do a good job but aren't as thorough as the RO systems.

Your body needs plenty of water for a successful pregnancy—after all, you and your baby are made of more than 60 percent water. Contaminated water makes everything more difficult for father, mother, and baby, whereas clean water fosters healthy life and growth.

Electromagnetic Fields

Electromagnetic fields (EMFs) are produced by electric lines, cell phones, wireless devices, WiFi access points, microwave ovens, and pretty much anything powered with electricity. Here we explain how EMFs affect our bodies, where they come from, and what to do about them. There's convincing evidence that some EMFs are harmful. Since there's zero risk to reducing EMF levels, it's worth doing.

There's more than a century of medical research supporting the idea that our bodies are both chemical and electrical. Robert Becker, a physician formerly with the Veterans Administration in Syracuse, New York, who spent his career researching how the body relates to electricity, and demonstrated that the body's electrical fields help the stem cells in a growing fetus to "know" how to differentiate and become different types of cells. When we learned how easily cells responded to electrical fields, we thought it best to allow the natural electrical currents in Lana's body to influence the development of our children instead of the EMFs from the electronic devices around her.

Long-term exposure to EMFs has been linked to cancer, chromosome damage in babies, infertility, and miscarriage. Studies show that women exposed to EMF levels at levels commonly found near household wiring (1.6 microtesla or greater) were nearly twice as likely to miscarry as women not exposed to such strong fields. Minor reactions include headaches, dizziness, insomnia, fatigue, and depression.

One of Lana's medical associates, Dietrich Klinghardt, M.D., in Seattle, Washington, is known widely for his treatment of autism and other neurological conditions. Dr. Klinghardt is convinced that EMF exposure is tied directly to autism, and he even performed a small study in 2007 that showed that autism can be predicted based on the EMF levels of a pregnant mother's sleeping quarters. He concluded that pregnant women who sleep in areas with strong EMFs have children who are more likely to have neurological abnormalities, including autism, hyperactivity, and learning disorders.

In March 2008, a study was conducted in three Minnesota schools. In some classrooms, special filters were installed that reduced EMFs by more than 90 percent. Teachers filled out daily questionnaires about how they felt and about student behavior. In the reduced-EMF areas, teachers reported fewer headaches, asthma symptoms, and skin irritations. They felt more energetic and experienced less depression and anxiety, and elementary and middle school student behavior improved.

CAT scans, MRIs, ultrasounds, and X-rays expose people to significant EMF radiation. CAT scans present the highest risk, at 40 to 100 times the radiation of conventional X-rays. Ultrasounds of unborn babies are now routine. In May 2002, a study concluded, "There may be a relation between prenatal ultrasound exposure and adverse outcome." The observed effects of ultrasounds on a fetus have included growth restriction, delayed speech, dyslexia, damage to nerve myelin sheaths, and irreversible loss of brain cells.

Even so, most fetuses are exposed to ultrasounds and are still okay— but since our goal was maximum health, not just okay health, we chose to minimize the number of ultrasounds in each of our pregnancies, keeping it to one in the first trimester and one in the second. The first confirms that it is a normal pregnancy, and the second checks that all organs and limbs have formed properly.

If you are asked to have an ultrasound, we think it's smart to ask your provider, "What's the benefit?" The reasons for getting an ultrasound are usually weak, such as it being "routine" or "to help you bond with your baby." You'll bond with your baby anyway—mothers were bonding with their babies for thousands of years before the ultrasound was invented. The risk of a single ultrasound is low, but the risk of repeated ones is higher.

High-voltage transmission lines—the extra-tall power lines that run on pylon towers instead of poles—give off very strong EMFs—so if possible, don't live near them. The significant EMF exposure from high-voltage lines has been linked to child cancers and birth defects. If you already live near transmission lines and moving isn't an option, it's possible to install grounded metal shielding in your house for protection.

Cell phones are another source of EMFs. In 1998, retired electrical engineer Lloyd Morgan of the Central Brain Tumor Registry, found out he had a brain tumor. His neurosurgeon told him that EMF exposure was a possible cause. Morgan decided to explore the link between EMFs and brain tumors more carefully. He conducted a study that found that over-exposure to cell phone radiation can lead to brain tumors, DNA damage, and infertility, and his study has been endorsed by more than forty doctors and scientists.

Not many people know it, but cell phone user manuals warn customers to keep the cell phones away from their bodies, even when the phone is not in use. In one study, scientists reviewed eleven different reliable studies of people who had used cell phones for more than ten years, and they found that cell phone use approximately doubles the risk of getting brain cancer on the side of the head to which the cell phone was usually held.

We weren't about to go back to the dark ages and give up our cell phones and electronics, but we did reduce our exposure to extra EMFs. Here's the plan we devised, which we still follow today:

- When carrying a cell phone in a pocket, we either turn it off or put it on airplane mode if we're not expecting an immediate call. Airplane mode reduces the EMF output substantially. Lana carries the phone in her purse instead of her pocket. When using a cell phone, we put it on speakerphone whenever possible. If we need to make a private phone call, we use a wired headset. After a while this became habit and we didn't notice doing it anymore.

- Cordless landline phones emit a constant EMF field throughout the house. We thought this was one EMF source we could eliminate altogether, so we replaced our cordless phones with regular corded phones. We found high-quality phones with good speakerphones and headsets that work across the room.

- Given all of the findings on EMFs, as well as the changes created in proteins from the high heat, microwave ovens just don't seem worth the trouble. We use a halogen convection oven instead, which is nearly as fast as a microwave, makes better-tasting food, and is safer.

- We upgraded our computer monitors and televisions to LCD, LED, or plasma screens. The old screens emit far more EMFs. If we still had an older TV, we would stay four to five feet away from it.

- We never set our laptop computers on our laps or in direct contact with our bodies, and we try to use them on battery power, since they have a lot more EMF when plugged in. Lana never set her laptop on her lap while pregnant.

- We replaced our plug-in alarm clocks with battery-powered ones, or we moved a plug-in one four to five feet away from the head of our bed.

- Hair dryers use high frequencies to drive the motor quickly and produce heat. Lana didn't use a hair dryer during pregnancy unless she was in a hurry.

- We never keep an electric blanket on while we sleep.

- We installed an easy-to-reach on-off switch for our WiFi access point so we could turn it off when we weren't using it and while we slept. We also ran Ethernet cables to our desks for Internet access so we could keep the WiFi off while we worked at our computers for longer periods.

- We installed affordable plug-in EMF filters on some of the outlets in our house.

- We made sure that our bed and our baby's crib didn't contain metal. Metal picks up ambient EMFs in the room and conducts them.

- Lana stopped wearing bras that contain metal. Lots of women actually report feeling better from switching to metal-free bras.

Were we paranoid? Quite possibly. But we're certain the changes we made didn't introduce any *additional* risk, and there's ample evidence that they did lots of good. You don't have to do everything on this list to improve your pregnancy; even one thing, like the EMF filters listed on www.betterbabybook.com/emf, can have a big impact.

11

Endotoxins: The Toxins Produced inside You

Endotoxins are toxins produced inside our bodies either by our own cells or by the bacteria, fungi, and other microbes that live inside us. Because endotoxins are produced inside the body, we have to deal with them differently from toxins that come from the outside. For toxins that come from the outside, we do our best to avoid the source. For endotoxins, our goal is to help the body produce fewer and eliminate them as easily, quickly, and safely as possible.

People have lots of organisms living inside their bodies—trillions, in fact. Some of the organisms that live inside us are always harmful, like ringworm or flatworm parasites (not everyone has them, but many people do). Others, like the yeast *Candida albicans*, are always present in the body but can become a problem when they are allowed to grow and reach higher levels.

Many of the organisms help us. You wouldn't be healthy without the good probiotic bacteria in your GI tract. The word *probiotic* means "for life." These bacteria play an important role in digestion, and fight the harmful microbes in us. Without these little guys, your food wouldn't be nearly as useful to you, and harmful bacteria could flourish and promote disease.

Probiotic flora pass into newborn babies through mother's milk—so they're there to help you from the very beginning. About four pounds of your weight comes from gut flora alone, and the number of individual bacteria living in your gut far exceeds the number of cells in your body.

The harmful organisms that live inside us excrete waste just as people do. *Endotoxins* is really just a fancy word for this waste. Many people don't eliminate endotoxins as easily or as quickly as they should. This can result in symptoms ranging from annoying ailments to chronic diseases. Endotoxins create an environment in a mother's body that's not ideal for her own health or for a growing fetus's.

Our goal was to help Lana's body get rid of endotoxins before they reached our babies. In this section, we explain two scenarios that lead to higher endotoxin levels in a mother's body and describe what you can do to reverse the situation.

First, sometimes endotoxins remain inside the body and are not eliminated. We explain techniques that help the body to eliminate them. Second, sometimes endotoxins are produced too quickly for the body to handle. In this case, the answer is to help the body kill the harmful microbes that are producing the endotoxins—that is, treat the source (the harmful bacteria) and not the symptoms (the endotoxins). We explain how to get rid of harmful intruders, prevent them from returning, and make your body a safe, clean home for your baby.

The GI tract—the stomach, the small intestine, and the colon (or large intestine)—is one of body's main systems and comes into contact with the outside world every time we eat. We can't live without food, but sometimes food contains bacteria or fungi we don't want in our bodies. The GI tract usually does a great job of absorbing nutrients from foods and eliminating intruders.

Our probiotic gut flora help the GI tract by creating digestive enzymes and fighting intruders. They're central to the delicate balance in a healthy GI tract. Problems with endotoxins begin either when our probiotic flora population becomes weaker or when harmful intruders become too numerous for our probiotic flora to handle. Proper digestion is so important to health that Hippocrates, one of the first doctors in recorded history, said that "bad digestion is the root of all evil." Let's look at how bad digestion happens so we can make good digestion routine.

Intestinal imbalance occurs when the number, type, or location of intestinal flora is changed from its natural equilibrium. A variety of diseases and digestive problems are caused by intestinal imbalance. These include stomach pains, bloating, constipation, diarrhea, skin infections, itchy skin, eczema, psoriasis, acne, yeast infections, new food allergies, fatigue, brain fog, anxiety, mood swings, irritability, headaches, and intense craving for sugar. In extreme cases, diseases like irritable bowel syndrome, inflammatory bowel disease, or rheumatoid arthritis may develop.

These ailments are naturally stressful for a pregnant mother to deal with, so the result is that the fetus is exposed not only to higher levels of endotoxins but also to higher levels of stress hormones, both of which promote defense mode at the expense of growth. Let's look at two examples:

1. *Diarrhea.* Probiotic flora produce special fats in the intestines called short-chain fatty acids (SCFAs). These SCFAs are a central part of electrolyte and water absorption in the colon. Too few probiotic flora means fewer SCFAs. If the situation is extreme, electrolyte imbalance leads to water retention in the intestines, resulting in diarrhea. SCFAs improve colonic blood flow, increase the absorption of calcium and other nutrients, and are important for a healthy mucus lining in the colon. If your SCFA levels are low over time, you'll get fewer nutrients out of your food.

2. *Food allergies.* Any time your probiotic population decreases, the production of mucin, acidic mucopolysaccharides, and immunoglobulin decreases in the intestines. These molecules prevent harmful microbes from adhering to intestinal mucus, so lower levels of them means it's easier for pathogens to live in your GI tract. If harmful pathogens become too numerous in the intestines, the endotoxins they produce can break down the intestinal mucus lining. A weak intestinal lining allows large pieces of

undigested food to be absorbed into the bloodstream and distributed throughout the body. The immune system doesn't recognize these large molecules and sends antibodies to attack them. The result is that you become allergic to foods you used to tolerate. If this continues over a long period, autoimmune diseases can develop.

The most common causes of intestinal imbalance are antibiotics, stress, eating too much sugar, and consuming sulfites (common in our food supply).

Antibiotics kill the good bacteria along with the bad. Unfortunately, your probiotic population takes longer to recover than harmful microorganisms do. When the course of antibiotics is complete, harmful bacteria multiply and grow faster because they face less resistance from your now weakened probiotic population. Yeasts thrive the whole time because they're immune to antibiotics, and the probiotics that fight them have been weakened. The longer the dosage and the stronger the antibiotic, the worse it is for your probiotic population and the more likely it is to result in intestinal imbalance. Antibiotics result in weaker probiotic levels for months after the course is finished, so even infrequent use is harmful to gut balance. Antibiotics cure diseases and save lives, but it's important to take probiotics after using them.

Psychological stress also harms probiotics. The probiotic flora in young primates decreases when they're first separated from their mothers. Similarly, Soviet cosmonauts had low probiotic levels when they returned from stressful space travel. The decreased levels persisted for several days after their safe return to Earth. Stress also results in a sustained increase in our fight-or-flight hormones. These hormones make it easier for harmful microorganisms to thrive.

Harmful pathogens in the GI tract live on sugar and carbohydrates—especially *Candida*. When *Candida* has lots of food to eat, it overgrows easily. Using antibiotics while eating sugar is a prime recipe for *Candida* overgrowth: the antibiotic weakens the probiotic population while the *Candida* (a fungus) lives on, happily eating sugars and carbs. A diet too high in sugar and carbs can also slow down bowel transit time, giving food more time to ferment in the gut. Fermentation produces endotoxins.

Sulfur compounds—sulfates and sulfites—are used as preservatives in many of today's foods. Common examples are dried fruits, dehydrated vegetables, packaged fruit juices, baked goods, white bread, alcoholic beverages, and shellfish. When you eat these sulfur compounds, they increase the growth of potentially harmful pathogens in the GI tract. This happens because some kinds of gut bacteria change sulfur compounds into sulfide, which can damage the mucus lining of the intestinal wall. The weakened mucus lining allows harmful bacteria to grow more easily, resulting in intestinal imbalance.

Intestinal imbalance can also result from undigested protein passing into the colon. If this happens, the undigested protein can ferment and produce endotoxins before it's eliminated.

Here's a checklist for keeping a balanced GI tract:

- Probiotic supplements help to keep the GI tract in balance. Our website, www.betterbabybook.com/probiotics, contains a list of our favorite brands.

- Avoid using antibiotics if you can. If your doctor prescribes them, supplement with a higher dose of probiotics after the course is complete.

- Keep your stress level as low as possible, because stress kills your probiotic flora. We cover stress reduction in chapter 15.

- Eat a diet low in sugars and carbs. Chapters 4 and 5 talk all about diet and explain lots of other benefits of avoiding sugars and carbs.

- Avoid foods that contain sulfites and sulfates (see list above).

12

How to Deal with Toxins

Usually we try to avoid toxins. Endotoxins are a little different; we cannot really avoid them, because they're produced inside us. But we can do our best to stop them from being produced and to clean them out. Our bodies are great at eliminating toxins on their own, but there are lots of products that help us to detox faster and easier. Here are the substances we used during pregnancy.

Activated Charcoal

You'll find activated charcoal at your local pharmacy. It's used in poison control centers and emergency rooms worldwide because it's such an effective detoxifier. It's also used in air and water purifiers, kidney dialysis machines, and the like. Activated charcoal has been proved harmless even in large doses—it just passes through the GI tract. Activated charcoal is extremely porous inside and out. It can adsorb many times its own weight in toxins.

Adsorption is different from *absorption*. *Adsorb* means to actively capture something, whereas *absorb* means to passively soak something up. Activated charcoal adsorbs toxins, which means that it proactively seeks them out, captures them, and carries them out of the body. It adsorbs a majority of organic chemicals, many inorganic chemicals, and a variety of other toxins, including mycotoxins and endotoxins.

Activated charcoal adsorbs so much that if you take it with any prescription drug, it can almost neutralize the drug's effect. When you ingest activated charcoal, it purifies your digestive fluids, adsorbs toxins and drugs, prevents their reabsorption into your body, and decreases the liver's workload.

You'll find activated charcoal sold as powder, capsules, and tablets. We use the powder, and in the finest grade we can find (it's less gritty this way). The capsules don't contain much, so you have to take about twenty capsules to get one to two tablespoons of activated charcoal. Not only is taking twenty capsules a bit unpleasant, it also gets expensive.

For a general detox before pregnancy, we recommend anywhere between one teaspoon and one tablespoon of activated charcoal powder mixed with cool water one to three times per day on an empty stomach. You should do this for at least a month before getting pregnant. Using cool water is important, because if the water is hot, the charcoal will deactivate and lose a lot of its adsorptive power. While activated charcoal has almost no taste, it can be a little gritty and goes down more smoothly if you add bentonite clay, which we discuss next. Both of these can be constipating, so you may need more fiber or magnesium, too. Reduce or eliminate the dose until things are running smoothly.

While you are pregnant, we suggest taking a teaspoon of activated charcoal with any meal that contains the foods we recommended not to eat in chapter 4 or with anything else you know is unhealthy. The activated charcoal will help to keep the toxins in these foods away from your baby. There's no need to take activated charcoal daily while you're pregnant, but if you start to feel nauseous or get morning sickness symptoms like bloating, gas, vomiting, stiff joints, or a headache, one to two tablespoons on an empty stomach can help. During pregnancy, low levels of toxins can cause these symptoms. Using activated charcoal to relieve these symptoms during pregnancy is nothing new—it was mentioned as early as 1898 in *King's American Dispensatory*, a book first published in 1854 that covers the use of herbs used in American medical practice.

Bentonite Clay

Bentonite clay is a powerful detoxifier that has been used internally and externally throughout history. Bentonite is found throughout the Great Plains in the United States. Originally, it was formed from heat and volcanic activity, which instilled it with a negative electromagnetic charge.

When bentonite comes into contact with the water in your GI tract, it "awakens" as the water releases its negative charges and makes it highly porous and adsorptive, just like activated charcoal. This release stimulates a healing energy flow throughout the body as the clay attracts and adsorbs positively charged toxins and acts as a sponge absorbing others. Bentonite clay even adsorbs heavy metals, some mycotoxins (including aflatoxin), and some pesticides and herbicides. Since the clay is not assimilated into the body, any toxins it adsorbs or absorbs on its way through the GI tract leave with it. This eases the burden on the liver and kidneys.

Bentonite clay is one of the oldest, safest, and cheapest ways to detox. It has a mild, creamy, nondescript flavor. Like activated charcoal, it's best taken on an empty stomach. You'll find bentonite clay in liquid and powder forms. We use the liquid, because there's an ideal ratio of water to clay that makes the clay most effective, and liquid bentonite products are mixed at this ratio. Lana took one tablespoon of bentonite per day on an empty stomach before and during pregnancy. When she took it with charcoal, she took a lower dose of each to avoid constipation.

Chlorella

Chlorella is a microscopic algae that grows in fresh water. You take it as a supplement in little tablets. Chlorella works to repair nerve tissues (including the brain) and helps to prevent cancer. It enables probiotics to grow, promoting intestinal balance and reducing endotoxins. Finally, as a powerful natural chelator, chlorella helps the body to eliminate toxic heavy metals. It also aids in detoxifying the body from pesticides and herbicides.

When you buy chlorella, it's important to choose "broken cell wall" chlorella. Chlorella algae cells have strong cell walls, so if the walls aren't broken ahead of time, the chlorella typically passes right through the body without much benefit. We recommend taking twenty to thirty tablets daily for a month or two. After our initial cleanse, we just take chlorella when we eat seafood or think we might have been exposed to heavy metals.

Chlorella contains lots of iron. The body needs iron, but not too much. This means that chlorella is great to take as a temporary detox, but not all the time. For the same reason, don't take chlorella at the exact same time as vitamin C, because that would facilitate iron absorption.

Cholestyramine

Cholestyramine is one of the original drugs designed to lower choles-terol. Questran is a popular brand. Normally the liver excretes liver bile at the beginning of the small intestine, and the bile is reabsorbed at the end of the small intestine. Cholestyramine works to lower cholesterol by binding with bile acids and escorting them out of the body. Cholestyr-amine is also very good at binding with certain mycotoxins—especially fumonisin—and can help the body to eliminate them. Its ability to elim-inate liver bile from the body also makes it useful for removing remnants of harsher prescription drugs. Cholestyramine is a prescription drug, so you'll have to consult your physician to use it.

Drugs versus Supplements

Drugs, whether they're over the counter, prescription, social (such as nicotine and alcohol), or illicit (such as narcotics), are often toxic to the body. That's why the drug effects don't last forever—your body works to get rid of them, and when it does get rid of them, the effects disappear.

Supplements, in contrast, are often substances that you'll find in food sources, and the body has no special need to get rid of them. If the effects of a supplement wear off, it's because the body has used them up, not because they've been purposefully eliminated. Taken in proper amounts, supplements are usually helpful and ease the burden of select systems throughout the body.

Prescription and Over-the-Counter Drugs

Although modern drugs save lives and often make us more comfortable, many of them harm a growing fetus. Many drugs are contraindicated during pregnancy. We think it's best to avoid using nearly all drugs during pregnancy if possible. Merck, one of the largest international drug manufacturers, acknowledges on its website that "drugs, unless absolutely necessary, should not be used during pregnancy because many can harm the fetus." For example, antidepressants can elevate the risk of preterm birth.

We think drugs shouldn't be used right before pregnancy, either. They may linger in the body, cross the placenta, and have the same adverse effects on the fetus as though they were being used currently, though perhaps without the same degree of damage. One way or another, keeping drugs away from the fetus was a top priority for us. When it came to the lives and health of our children, we wanted to be conservative.

We've reproduced a list of drugs and their effects on pregnancy at www.betterbabybook.com/pharmadrugs. If you've taken or been otherwise exposed to the drugs on that list, the detox techniques we discussed can help to protect your baby. Activated charcoal is one of the most effective techniques for removing drugs from the body. Conveniently, it's also one of the cheapest and easiest.

Although it's important to keep drugs away from your baby, drugs can save lives, but always work with your physician when you start *or stop* taking prescription drugs.

Social and Illicit Drugs

Detoxing before and during pregnancy is critical if you've smoked tobacco, consumed alcohol excessively, or have used or been exposed to illicit drugs within a year of conception. The research supporting this is so thorough and so widely publicized that we won't rehash it here. All of the details are available at www.betterbabybook.com/drugs. Fortunately, the detox techniques we discuss in this book are just as good at removing social and illicit drugs from the body as they are at removing pharmaceutical drugs and other toxins.

Morning Sickness and Toxins

Morning sickness is one of the ways a woman's body protects her baby from toxins in food. When you don't eat toxins, you don't get as much morning sickness. We know that with pregnant animals (cows, pigs, horses, and chickens), "feed rejection" is caused by contaminated food, even if the contamination is below the level at which an animal can taste it. A wide range of toxins can cause morning sickness in pregnant women.

Toxins make everyone sick, but pregnant women are naturally more sensitive to toxins in order to protect their babies. This is a convenient mechanism, because babies are easily hurt by toxins. A Cornell University study tested whether morning sickness was a mechanism to protect the baby from toxins or whether it was caused by a conflict between the mother and the baby's need for nutrition. The researchers observed that morning sickness reduces miscarriage, is positively correlated with toxin levels in mother's diet, and is closely related to food cravings and aversions. They concluded that morning sickness was indeed protecting the baby.

Lana didn't get morning sickness during either pregnancy. We think this happened because she detoxified her body extensively before each pregnancy and ate foods that were at very low risk for contamination with toxins during both pregnancies.

PART FOUR

Preparing for Pregnancy and Birth

13

Detoxifying Your Body and Your Home

For the steps outlined in this chapter, we recommend starting three to six months before getting pregnant, if possible. Three months is typically enough for your diet to improve fertility, but six months is best for detoxing properly. Working with a physician will give you access to medical tests that measure your progress.

The Better Baby Diet

The diet we recommend is based on our own experience combined with countless nutrition and diet books and thousands of studies. Dave refined the principles behind the diet for more than ten years—he used an early version of these principles in his twenties to lose a hundred pounds and improve his health. Lana used them to overcome nagging health problems. After two successful pregnancies, we have road-tested the diet with brilliant success. The Better Baby diet itself does wonders to detox the body. Starting it three to six months before getting pregnant is a firm foundation for your other detox efforts.

Heavy Metals and Chelation

By heavy metals, we mean metals that are toxic to the body. Examples are aluminum, arsenic, cadmium, chromium, copper, iron, mercury, manganese, nickel, and lead. People are exposed to heavy metals through food, dental fillings, cigarette smoke, air and water pollution, and some work environments. When these metals build up in our bodies over time, they can cause health problems. The body actually needs trace amounts of some metals, like copper and chromium. Other metals, like arsenic and mercury, only do harm.

At home, metals are most commonly found in tap water and certain foods. Tap water can become contaminated from old metal water pipes (lead, copper, and arsenic are all commonly found in old metal water pipes) or from contaminated local soil. Soil contamination usually happens near factories. Heavy metals are also contained in compact fluorescent lightbulbs and in household insecticides, fungicides, and rodenticides. Vaccines contain heavy metals as a preservative or an adjuvant (a substance that enhances the immune response).

Common food sources of heavy metals are factory-farmed chicken, eggs, and some pork products because of the use of antibiotics containing arsenic. Mercury contamination in seafood is now common, as we noted in chapter 4. Wild game hunted with lead shot or bullets is a risk, too. If you derive a lot of your diet from game, steel or bismuth shot is a healthier choice. Some pesticides contain lead, so its important to know where your vegetables come from, too.

Heavy metals are one reason that losing weight before *but not during* pregnancy is important. The body stores metals in fat deposits in order to keep the metals away from the more easily damaged organs and tissues. All methods of eliminating metals from the body stir them up from fat reserves, which prepares them for elimination. When you exercise, burn fat, and lose weight, any metals stored in the fat reserves that were burned will be released and will travel through the body. Some of the metals will be filtered out by the kidneys and the liver and eliminated, but some are likely to become deposited somewhere else in the body. This poses a risk for a fetus. Because of this, it's actually safer to keep the weight on along with the metals the fat is storing. This is one reason you shouldn't try to lose weight quickly while breastfeeding.

Chelation is a medical process that helps the body to detoxify from heavy metals. The process of chelation frees the metals from the fat reserves by breaking the chemical bonds between the two. Whenever you consume chelating foods, supplements, or drugs, they pull the heavy metals out of the fat deposits and release them into the bloodstream for filtration by the liver or the kidneys. Good chelators are alpha-lipoic acid, dimercaptosuccinic acid (DMSA), dimercaptopropane sulfonate (DMPS), and EDTA. DMPS is available only by prescription.

Once the chelators release the metals into the bloodstream, it's important to help the liver and the kidneys capture the metals using metal-cleansing supplements like dietary fiber, N-acetyl-cysteine, or chlorella. These supplements bind with the metals and carry them out of the body. Chelators alone simply dislodge the metals from the fat reserves and leave elimination up to the body. Sometimes, if there aren't enough cleansers circulating in the body, the heavy metals are simply redeposited in the body instead of eliminated. Like losing weight, strong chelation is important to avoid during pregnancy. When the chelators release the metals from the fat deposits, the risk that some of the metals will reach the fetus is too high. The ideal time to chelate is a full six months before pregnancy.

When dealing with heavy metals and chelation, we believe it's best to work with a holistic physician. Poorly implemented chelation can make you very sick and harm your liver and kidneys. DMSA and DMPS are usually administered orally and work best on chelating mercury. EDTA, which works best on lead, can be administered orally, but little is absorbed, so it's best administered through suppositories or intravenously. Chelation for serious cases of heavy metal toxicity usually involves intravenous administration of EDTA.

Great metal cleansers to take with these chelators are bentonite clay, chlorella, glutathione, N-acetyl-cysteine, and zeolite clay; most of these are mentioned throughout this book. Cilantro, a common spice, is also a wonderfully gentle chelator that cleanses the brain.

Rejuvenating Your Liver

Your liver is responsible for dealing with the toxins and chemicals we ingest (through food and drugs) and breathe in every day. Nearly a third of your blood is pumped through your liver every minute. As blood moves through the liver, the liver filters out harmful substances and neutralizes them. It also performs a number of other functions, including protein and hormone production, bile production, blood sugar (glucose) regulation and storage, and cholesterol and tryglyceride production. Without the liver, the body would die. An amazing organ, the liver is the only one that can regenerate itself.

We encounter preservatives, solvents, herbicides, pesticides, tobacco smoke, alcohol, heavy metals, and mycotoxins every day. Taking extra steps to help the liver detoxify the body keeps us healthy and prevents these toxins from reaching a growing fetus. Activated charcoal, bentonite and zeolite clays, and other detoxifiers bind toxins in the intestines and prevent them from ever reaching the liver. We highly recommend them.

Beyond these, there are herbs and supplements that optimize liver function so the body is prepared for what does get through. No matter how much activated charcoal or bentonite clay you use, many toxins will still get through to the liver. Vitamin C, N-acetyl-cysteine, and alpha-lipoic acid help to clean the liver's detoxification pathways. Silymarin, a powerful detoxifier found in milk thistle, has been shown to increase the liver's glutathione level as much as 35 percent, protect liver cells from the dangerous toxins they work with so closely, and stimulate liver regeneration. Artichoke extract has shown an ability to clean and protect the liver. Turmeric, hailed as one of the greatest herbs by ayurvedic medicine, can help the body to naturally increase liver bile flow, which enhances liver function and cleanses the liver.

We've found herbalist Hulda Clark's olive oil, grapefruit, and Epsom salt liver cleanse to be a great way to eliminate liver toxins from the body. We've both done the cleanse many times, and we always feel much better after doing it. You'll find a full description of this simple liver cleanse process on our website, www.betterbabybook.com/liver. We recommend doing this liver cleanse before *but not during* pregnancy.

Detoxifying Your Home

The best principle to remember when you're dealing with anything that you breathe or anything that comes in contact with your body is that if you cannot safely eat it, you should not inhale it or let it touch your skin. Your lungs quickly absorb particles in the air into your bloodstream, so any toxic chemical–containing fumes can be harmful. At the microscopic level your skin is a fine mesh, or net, and anything small enough will pass right through it and into your body. The molecules of chemicals, including those contained in the household products we discuss below, are often small enough to absorb through the skin.

Our goal in this section is to point out unexpected sources of toxins throughout your home. Of course, toxic poisons from expected sources—drain opener, toilet bowl cleaner, lawn chemicals, insecticides, pesticides, gasoline, lead paint, asbestos, toxic wood preservatives, or anything remotely like them—should be avoided completely if you are trying to get pregnant, are pregnant, or are nursing. Before conception, this goes for fathers, too. Every chemical you're exposed to right before and during pregnancy is likely to contact your baby. Spray chemicals are the easiest to be exposed to from normal use.

The Kitchen

Let's start with the kitchen, where we find dishwashing liquid, hand soap, dishwasher detergent, and probably some surface cleaners.

Artificial Fragrances

One health risk that many kitchen cleaning products have in common is the strong artificial fragrances they contain. These artificial fragrances consist of a variety of toxic estrogenic chemicals that are easily absorbed into the body when they are inhaled or touch your skin.

Skin contact, inhalation, or ingestion of the chemicals used in artificial fragrances will never fail to harm your body in some way. This is true no matter how low the concentration is or how "safe" the manufacturer, the FDA, or anyone else says these substances are. Artificial fragrances are harmful even when the concentration is low because toxic chemicals build up in the body over time and cause problems later. When you use these products every day, the chemicals can build up inside you.

One reason fragrances are toxic is that they contain oil-soluble molecules called *phthalates*. Have you ever noticed how strong fragrances are able to hang in the air for a long time? That unnatural, long-lasting smell lingers because phthalates, like oils, are difficult to break down— and they don't break down any faster in your lungs and bloodstream after you breath them in. There are a host of studies linking phthalates to birth complications.

The answer here is simple: use fragrance-free products.

Anything Made of Plastic

Plastic is a common source of toxins in the kitchen. This includes plastic cookware, dishes, silverware, storage containers, and disposable "paper" or styrofoam products, most of which are coated with plastic resin. Plastic or styrofoam articles that come into contact with your food or beverages often leach into the food or drink, and they're made from petrochemicals and dangerous substances like bisphenol-A (BPA). BPA is found in thousands of everyday consumer products, like canned foods (the lining inside the can), toilet paper, plastic cups, and recycled paper products.

BPA is a proven hormone disrupter that mimics estrogen in the body. Since BPA is a synthetic hormone, trace amounts have very different effects than do larger amounts, which have traditionally been considered toxic. In the 1970s and 1980s, scientists tested BPA and found that toxic levels caused organ failure and leukemia. These effects weren't seen when nontoxic levels were administered, so the chemical was considered safe. But later findings suggested that smaller amounts had very different yet still harmful effects.

BPA is released into hot foods and drinks (especially microwaved) very fast, so it's especially important to avoid hot food or drinks that have contacted plastic or Styrofoam. For example, one of the worst things you could do is something we see people in the workplace doing all the time: taking a Styrofoam cup of cold coffee and heating it in a microwave. The microwave is heating the BPA in the Styrofoam into the coffee, which people then drink.

To avoid BPA, we do the following:

- Avoid skin contact with vinyl.

- Drink bottled water only if it's bottled in glass.

- Avoid most canned foods and drinks, because a plastic epoxy resin lines the inside of the can.

- Don't microwave food in plastic containers or bags.

- Use glass or ceramic dishes and cups for dining, glass or ceramic containers for food storage, and stainless steel or wooden utensils.

- Buy fabric baby toys without chemical fire retardants instead of plastic ones.

Nonstick or Aluminum Cookware

Teflon, T-Fal, or any nonstick coated pans, pots, and other cookware contain fluoride compounds. When we discuss toothpaste a little later, we'll talk about why fluoride is dangerous. For now, you should know that when high heat is applied to these pans, these fluoride compounds and other harmful chemicals in the nonstick coatings are vaporizing into the air and leaching into your food.

This also happens with aluminum or aluminum-coated cookware. When this cookware is heated, harmful metallic aluminum ions leach into your food. Like fluoride, aluminum has been proven to cause health problems.

Stainless steel and cast iron are pretty safe, but high heat still releases the metal ions into food. Glass, enameled, or ceramic cookware is best. Ceramic is by far the most convenient: unlike glass, it's resistant to cracking even when subjected to fast temperature changes. Good ceramic cookware can be heated to over 2,000 degrees Fahrenheit without cracking. It also has a relatively nonstick surface, won't scratch, and is pretty lightweight. You can't throw ceramic around, however, because a heavy impact can crack it.

The Laundry Room

Fragrances are also one of the main sources of toxins in your laundry room, where we find detergent, softener, and bleach. Standard laundry detergents and softeners have chemicals and fragrances in them that are especially strong and are designed to linger in clothing for days. Before Lana became pregnant, we switched to fragrance-free laundry detergent and stopped using fabric softeners.

Dryer sheets are the worst culprit in this category. When you use a dryer sheet, your clothing is coated with powerful artificial chemicals that are absorbed through the skin. When you put these clothes on, the toxins are absorbed through your skin and into your bloodstream, especially when you sweat and water mixes with the chemical residue on the clothing. We have not used dryer sheets for many years.

When choosing a bleach, go with oxygen bleach; it is much safer to use than standard chlorine bleach. Chlorine bleach fumes are toxic. We all know the strong smell of chlorine bleach—it really gets your attention. If you're breathing in the fumes, they are surely reaching your baby. Oxygen bleach is a great alternative that emits few fumes at all, it removes stains and odors well, and it won't ruin colored clothing.

New clothes, towels, sheets, and the like come with fragrance and chemicals from the manufacturing process. They can also be infused with nanosilver particles as a preservative. If you've ever bought a shirt and put it on right away, you might notice a bit of skin irritation—this is why. The first thing we do when we buy new clothes or household textile products is to wash them in oxygen bleach or 20 Mule Team Borax (boric acid) before using them. This removes the chemicals and nanosilver before they touch your body.

The Bathroom

The bathroom contains personal hygiene products and cosmetics such as shampoo, soap, toothpaste, deodorant, perfumes and colognes, makeup, hair dye, shaving cream, and hair spray or styling gel. Almost all of these products contain artificial fragrances (especially perfumes and colognes). The same principle applies here: natural or fragrance-free products are safer for your baby.

In contrast to dishwasher detergent or laundry detergent, personal care products come in close and prolonged contact with your skin and lungs every day. We're going to discuss a few of these products individually, but first we'd like to point out two common chemicals to avoid that you'll find in many personal care products: sodium laureth sulfate and parabens. Then we'll discuss toothpaste, deodorant, perfume, makeup, hair dye, sunscreen, other toiletries, and baby products.

Sodium Laureth Sulfate

Sodium laureth sulfate (SLS) and its close relative sodium lauryl sulfate and their cousins are used as foaming agents. They're common in toothpaste, shampoo, and soap. SLS is a corrosive chemical used to dissolve grease on car engines and garage floors, among other industrial uses. Even though SLS might make your shampoo or toothpaste foam up nicely, we've known since 1983 that SLS is toxic and can cause irritation even in small amounts. It's also another hormone disrupter (like BPA) that mimics estrogen. As such, it can contribute to premenstrual syndrome, menopausal symptoms, male infertility, and breast cancer. Lots of companies maintain that they use safe amounts of SLS—we don't agree with them. The safest amount of SLS is none.

Parabens

Parabens are antifungal preservatives found in skin and face creams. Parabens were found in more than 13,200 products in 1984. They are easily absorbed into the bloodstream through the skin. Mainstream science has long held that they are harmless and rapidly eliminated from the body, but we found recent evidence that parabens have been linked to breast cancer and hormone disruption. Ingredient names to watch out for are methylparaben, ethylparaben, propylparaben, butylparaben, isobutyl-paraben, and E216.

Toothpaste

Since toothpaste goes in your mouth, plenty of it gets into your bloodstream, even if you don't swallow any. When choosing a toothpaste that's safe, you'll want one that is free of fluoride, SLS, and titanium dioxide.

For years fluoride has been advertised as a benefit in toothpaste, but it turns out that fluoride is dangerous for people—it's even more toxic than lead. Fluoride poisoning severely weakens bones, and there's evidence that it actually makes tooth enamel more porous and teeth *more* susceptible to decay over time.

The problem with fluoride in toothpaste is that it builds up in the body over time, so even the trace amounts in toothpaste are harmful after years of use. The kidneys can filter out only about 50 percent of one's total fluoride intake. In 1977, the National Academy of Sciences reported that an average person who consumed two milligrams of fluoride per day for forty years would contract crippling skeletal fluorosis, which damages joints and bones, by the end of that period. A 1995 study concluded that fluoride leads to lower IQ in children. Doses of fluoride as low as 0.1 to 0.3 milligrams per kilogram, well below the levels in toothpaste, can cause symptoms of fluoride toxicity, including gastrointestinal pain, nausea, vomiting, and fever.

Aside from being in toothpaste, fluoride is added to mouthwash and even some drinking water. There are fluoride pills and fluoride treatments at the dentist's office. In the name of preventing tooth decay, some pediatricians really do recommend giving sodium fluoride pills to your children. We wonder if they know that industrial fluoride containers are marked with a skull and crossbones. On January 20, 1979, the *New York Times* reported a $750,000 settlement received by parents of a three-year-old child killed by fluoride in the dental chair.

Deodorant and Antiperspirant

Commercial deodorants typically contain artificial fragrances. When the high amount of sweat in the underarm area mixes with this fragrance, the harmful chemicals in the fragrance are easily absorbed into the body.

Antiperspirants contain forms of aluminum, typically aluminum oxide, and that's how they work. Aluminum oxide is a potent astringent that closes the pores and stops you from sweating. It works pretty well if that's your goal. The problem with this is that the armpit is a central lymph area where the body seeks to eliminate toxins by sweating. If you prevent sweating in that area, the toxins that would have been eliminated are pushed back into the body (right near the lymph nodes). Not only is this unhealthy, it is usually occurring on a daily basis with almost no break at all. Furthermore, aluminum itself is toxic and has been linked with respiratory and neurological problems.

Many people have tried natural deodorants and complain that they don't work. We have a surprise for you: you'll probably find that when you detox and eat the low-sugar diet we describe in this book, underarm body odor will start to decrease on its own, and your need for strong artificial deodorants and antiperspirants will decrease. As always, the health of the outside of your body tells you how things are going on the inside.

Perfume, Cologne, and Eau de Toilette

Have you ever felt a bit queasy when someone wearing too much perfume entered the room? Most of us have. Designer fragrances are made of neurotoxic chemicals made from petroleum products. They're made to linger in the air and on clothes for months. Petroleum chemicals typically make up 80 to 90 percent of a bottle of perfume. It's a good idea to avoid fragrances during pregnancy. Even secondhand exposure is a bad idea. It's so well-known that fragrances make people sick that they're frequently banned in schools, hospitals, and offices.

Makeup

Makeup often contains parabens, SLS, heavy metals, and other toxins. Blush often contains propylene glycol (antifreeze), which is known to produce allergic reactions. A 2007 study found that up to one-third of lipsticks contain lead in amounts above the FDA limit. Lip glosses frequently contain toxic fragrance, which in this case is not just inhaled but eaten in trace amounts on a daily basis year after year. In forty-five years, a user is likely to swallow two pounds of lipstick or lip gloss. Mascara usually contains parabens. Nail polish contains toluene, which can affect the kidneys, the liver, and the heart. Formaldehyde is also an ingredient in the hardeners used in nail polish. Nail polish remover contains acetone, a known toxic irritant.

Since makeup sits on the skin all day, it seeps through the pores and into the bloodstream, especially if it mixes with sweat. It's best to avoid any makeup that is not natural and organic, especially during pregnancy. Remember: if you can't eat it, it shouldn't be touching your skin. This goes especially for products like makeup that have prolonged contact with the skin day after day.

Hair Dye

Hair dye often contains toxins like acetate, ammonia, coal tar, parabens, pthalates, and SLS. Women who dye their hair are exposed to these chemicals soaking into their scalps for hours every four to six weeks for years. Stylists who come into contact with the dyes day after day are especially at risk. Studies have shown that black hair dye is the most harmful because it contains harsher chemicals and sometimes toxic metals.

It's wise to avoid using hair dye altogether or to use one of the few safe brands free of toxic chemicals. We list those on www.betterbaby-book.com/hair. At a minimum, if you use a toxic hair die, use it in such a way that it doesn't come in contact with the scalp. Some doctors recommend refraining from hair dye during the first trimester. But if not during the first trimester, then why during the second or third or while nursing? These chemicals build up in the body and the brain over time. A little now, a little in six weeks, and a little more six weeks after that turns into a lot over ten years.

Sunscreen

Sunscreen and sunblock lotion sometimes contain estrogen hormone disrupters like camphor. Many of these products also contain titanium dioxide as the active ingredient. Titanium dioxide is a harmful metal that is sometimes used as a white dye in products like toothpaste and food coloring. Many sunblock lotions use the nanoparticulate form of titanium dioxide. The nanoparticulate form is made of very small molecules that are easily absorbed through the skin and can cross the placenta and even penetrate into individual cells in the body.

Although using sunscreen might be safer than getting a bad sunburn, it is far healthier to expose your skin to the sun every day you're pregnant, right up to the point before you get a light burn. This lets your body make the most active form of vitamin D3 called vitamin D sulfate. Supplements do not create this form of D3. In addition, the only form of cholesterol that can cross the placenta to form a baby's growing brain is cholesterol sulfate, which is formed when you expose your skin to sunlight. A lack of sunlight will limit the amount of tissue building blocks your baby gets. One theory ties a lack of sunlight in mothers with a higher risk of autism. It is simply a bad idea to avoid the sun or wear sunscreen when you're pregnant.

Other Toiletries

Shaving cream usually contains parabens, but it also contains a chemical called DEHA, which is known to cause cancerous tumors in mice. Many body soaps contain propylene glycol, which is easily absorbed through the skin and can depress the nervous system. Antidandruff shampoos that contain zinc pyrithone might be a risk, too—rats given zinc pyrithone for two weeks developed deformities. Considering that hair sprays are breathed in during application and sit on the scalp for hours thereafter, we couldn't find a safe one that actually worked.

Baby Products

Baby products, including diaper cream and sunscreen, often contain more than twenty-seven chemicals that aren't proven safe for babies. Diaper cream can contain sodium borate, and sunscreen contains oxybenzone, two toxic chemicals that can accumulate in a baby's body and have adverse effects. Oxybenzone is an endocrine disruptor that could cause imbalance in a young baby's hormone system. We made sure that everything contacting our baby's skin was natural and chemical-free. If we didn't know what all of the ingredients were in a product, we didn't use it. Our kids get a reasonable amount of sunshine on bare skin, then put on the most natural sunscreen of all, a shirt and a hat.

Shower Curtains

Vinyl shower curtains are a big source of estrogenic chemicals in bathrooms. Select polyester instead.

The Garage, the Basement, and Other Rooms

Gasoline, diesel, kerosene, fuel oil, pesticides, herbicides, fertilizers like Miracle Grow, weed killers like Round-Up, strong cleaning chemicals, hand soaps, and the like are all toxic and can produce toxic fumes. It's best to store them in a shed or a structure that is not connected to your immediate living area.

Carbon monoxide is a deadly odorless gas and a by-product of fire, so any type of gas stove, heater, car exhaust, or burning device can produce it. The easy solution to carbon monoxide is to install detectors in your home. If you have a basement with cracked walls or floors, it's a good idea to check for radon, another toxic odorless gas that forms from uranium in soil and rock.

Common household items like carpets and even some furniture and bedding contain poisonous chemicals and fire retardants that give off gas over time into the air you breathe. New paint and furniture anywhere in the house can raise the level of toxins in your circulating air. Pay particular attention to buying nontoxic furniture.

If these articles burn, they release enormous amounts of toxins. Breathing in just a small amount of this type of smoke from a house fire could be devastating for your fetus, so smoke detectors are also part of making a nontoxic home.

Fluoride lurks not just in toothpaste and nonstick cookware like teflon and T-Fal but also in microwave popcorn bags and stain-guarded clothing, furniture, and carpets.

Most of us have heard a lot about lead poisoning but may not be familiar with all of its sources. It's a good idea to check older pipes (your water supply), paints and imported miniblinds (air quality), and crystal dishes (your food). Lots of decorative crystal dishes are made of leaded glass that transfers lead into your food.

You may think that you're far away from these chemicals, but we encourage you to double-check. In 2004, researchers found traces of cosmetics, pesticides, gasoline, garbage, and burned coal in the umbilical cords of ten newborn babies they tested.

Avoid Cat Litter

Studies have shown that it's important for pregnant women to avoid cat feces. The reason is that a strain of bacteria called *Toxoplasma gondii* is excreted in cat feces. If a pregnant woman contracts *T. gondii*, this bacteria can result in severe health problems for the developing fetus. If you have cats, it's important to avoid cleaning their litter box while you're pregnant. It's also important to get your cat tested and treated if necessary before you get pregnant. Indoor cats that don't catch mice and birds are at much lower risk. We even recommend using gloves when gardening and thoroughly washing any garden vegetables if you have a problem with stray cats using your garden as a litter box.

Do Your Best

Even though toxic chemicals abound in our modern society, millions of healthy children are born every year in spite of their exposure to these chemicals. We took the steps described here because it made sense, but we didn't obsess about what we couldn't control. The only thing we can do is our best!

To learn about the exact products we used during our pregnancies, visit www.betterbabybook.com/household.

14

Autism

As you may have heard on the news, autism is a fast-growing health problem in the United States and around the world. Data reported in 2007 indicated that one in ninety-one children in the United States is diagnosed with an autism spectrum disorder. This means that more than 1 percent of our children have it. Almost 2 percent of our boys have it. The concern has been widely publicized as people around the country and the world search for causes so they can treat autistic kids and avoid autism in the future.

The debate about the cause of autism is charged with emotion and controversy because it has a big effect on families, and some companies could face liability claims larger than those from asbestos if certain materials are identified as causal factors. Although some physicians are very supportive of our approach to autism, there are others who believe that autism is caused by genetics only. We know that autism is related to each of the risk factors we mention, but there are few studies showing that avoiding those risk factors will result in autism-free children. We started at a higher risk level for having an autistic child, because Lana was almost forty and Dave has a family history of a mild form of autism called Asperger's syndrome, but by using our plan we were able to avoid autism in our children.

In fact, Dave grew up with many symptoms of Asperger's and ADHD before discovering the biochemistry behind his symptoms and reversing them years ago. For us as parents, avoiding autism was personal and motivated a lot of our early research. For our children, we wanted to eliminate anything and everything that might raise our risk. As scientists and researchers grounded in the real world, we know that it's nearly impossible to remove all risk, but we wanted to reduce it as much as we could.

We believe our program has a very high likelihood of reducing the risk of autism because it supports healthy immune function and reduces unhealthy inflammation, ensures proper nutritional intake, and avoids and eliminates toxins that are associated with autism risk. We are certain there is no single cause for every case of autism, but we believe that autism can—and has been—cured many times, and we believe it can be avoided by a prudent application of the principles outlined in our book. That said, although there are many studies supporting our recommendations, there is no double-blind study of our program in its entirety. We welcome the opportunity to conduct one, however.

After the research we conducted, and based on Lana's work as the medical director of a lab testing company interacting with integrative physicians across the country, we concluded that there are many triggers for autism but that in most cases it manifests as a neuroinflammatory condition affecting the myelin sheath of a baby's neurons.

We highlight the risk factors for autism in the following sections, and we cite our research each time so you can measure the strength of our conclusions for yourself.

Possible Causes of Autism

We have found that autism can be brought on by toxic heavy metals, older parents, exposure to toxins in the womb (especially mycotoxins from molds), a stressful womb environment triggering changes in the sympathetic nervous system, some genetically modified foods, morphinelike substances in wheat and dairy, too much iron, vitamin D deficiency, and an imbalance in probiotics in the digestive tract. There is even some surprising—and potentially scary—early research indicating that electromagnetic frequency (EMF) radiation and fluorescent lighting may slightly increase the risks, and we know with certainty that these make some autism spectrum conditions worse. More research is needed here. CFL and fluorescent lights do not help people be healthier and may cause harm.

Even some elements of a baby's birth experience, like early cutting of the umbilical cord or inadequate contact with the mother in the first few minutes of life, can heighten the risk of autism, probably by triggering changes in the sympathetic nervous system. There is also a nutritional risk from a poor infant diet (lack of breastfeeding), and there seems to be a genetic risk linked to our ability to excrete toxins.

This is such a long list of possible causes that it's no surprise there is an emotional and confusing debate about autism. In our experience, autism manifests when a combination of these risk factors sets up a child's immune system to overreact to certain environmental triggers.

In this chapter, we show how the recommendations in this book can protect a baby from autism as it's currently understood. We focus on what you can do while you're pregnant—or better yet, while you're planning to get pregnant—to lower the risk of autism.

Heavy Metals

Heavy metals—including aluminum, lead, arsenic, cadmium, and especially mercury—have been linked to autism. The sources of heavy metals in daily life include cigarette smoke, seafood, dental fillings and bridgework, vaccines, and toxic metal vapor in some workplaces.

If you're a smoker, we know you've heard this before, but stopping now before you even conceive might just reduce the risk of autism for your baby. Sticking to the safe seafood listed in chapters 4 and 5 allows you to enjoy seafood while avoiding heavy metals. If you have dental work like amalgam fillings, you might consult with a holistic dentist about having them removed and replaced at least three months before becoming pregnant. If you're pregnant and have metal fillings, do not make the mistake of having your fillings removed. Wait until you're done nursing to do it.

Vaccines are a controversial issue, but the truth is that some vaccines still do contain thimerosal (mercury). Many that don't have thimerosal contain aluminum salts as an adjuvant. It's best to research each vaccine yourself and consult with a holistic physician. Our purpose here is just to tell you that many vaccines do contain heavy metals, and heavy metals—and vaccines in general—are risk factors. If you do choose to vaccinate for flu or travel, following our heavy-metal detox regimen in chapter 13 will help. Evidence does not support the flu vaccine's efficacy compared to supplementing with vitamin D3.

Finally, if you're at risk for exposure to heavy metals in the workplace, you might seek a safer work environment before and during pregnancy. If that's not possible, strictly following all of the safety protocols is sure to help.

Age

Older parents do give birth to autistic children more frequently than younger parents do. Believe it or not, this is especially true of older fathers. We know there's no way to get younger, but there are a number of steps both men and women can take to improve reproductive function and sperm quality. Chapter 13 is loaded with information about detoxing. The exercises in chapter 15 will also help to rejuvenate your body and its ability to reproduce. And the same foods and supplements described in chapters 5 and 7 that help a baby's genes be their best also help older parents to have healthy eggs and sperm. We demonstrated that by following all the tips we've mentioned right here, it's possible for older parents with risk factors to have healthy kids.

Toxins

Keeping toxins away from your baby in the womb is essential, and several of the causes of autism we identified fall into this category. Mycotoxins from trace amounts of mold are particularly potent and harmful. Genetically modified foods have been directly linked to autism,

and so have the neurotoxins found in wheat and pasteurized milk products. Avoiding wheat and dairy has even become a mainstream method
for reducing autism symptoms in autistic children. We thought it made
sense to avoid these foods while our babies were in the womb, too, especially because wheat and dairy are carriers for common mycotoxins.

Some researchers even suspect that EMF exposure from cell phones
and electronics might contribute to autism, especially if these devices are
in a pregnant mother's sleeping quarters or held against her body while
she's pregnant. In fact, one shocking (but small) study was able to use
the EMF levels of a mother's bedroom during pregnancy to predict the
occurrence of autism later. The X-ray and microwave radiation emitted
from fluorescent lighting has also been hypothesized to be a contributing
factor. All of these toxins (or unnatural sources of radiation) may alter
the womb environment and send a fetus's epigenetic program into a
defensive mode, depriving the baby of critical growth opportunities.

GI Tract Imbalance

Nutritional imbalances that contribute to autism include gut dysbiosis.
Gut dysbiosis is an intestinal imbalance that results in unfriendly bacteria
in the gut causing elevated levels of endotoxins (toxins produced inside
the body). In a pregnant mother, these toxins can disrupt an unborn
baby's epigenetic program. Incidentally, gut dysbiosis in young children
has been linked to late-onset autism. Excess iron has been suspected; this
is important to know because iron supplements are very popular among
pregnant women. In our section on iron in chapter 7, we describe how to
reach the right balance of iron instead of having too little or too much.

Vitamin D3 Deficiency

A deficiency in vitamin D3 might turn out to be one of the biggest causes
of autism. Vitamin D3 is a hormone building block that protects a baby's
nerves and brain cells from many of the toxins and threats we've discussed. Although we knew it was important to avoid the risk factors for
autism we've mentioned, we recognized that it's nearly impossible to
avoid them completely. That's where taking plenty of vitamin D3 comes

in. Vitamin D3 protects your baby's brain from the small amount of exposure that is inevitable for all of us. Taking vitamin D3 is one of the cheapest and easiest things we recommend in this book, and it happens to be one of the most effective.

Keep Up with the Information

The same aspects of our program that boost fertility and help your baby to stay in growth mode also guard against the suspected causes of autism. We designed our program that way from the very beginning. But we aren't the first ones to say this: changing conditions bring about a constant need to update the information one needs to be healthy. Here we've done our best to provide the latest research on avoiding autism. This protocol worked for us, and we think it can reduce your risk as well. New information on preventing autism will be posted on our website, www .betterbabybook.com/autism, the moment we find out about it!

15

Reducing Stress
for an Easier and
Better Pregnancy

In addition to a special diet and detox protocols, reducing stress is good to do for fertility or pregnancy. For us and for most people, this is the hardest part of preparing for pregnancy and being pregnant. It's tougher, because it's not so black and white. A diet can be as simple as "eat this, don't eat that." But reducing stress takes psychological and emotional intention, and much of the time we aren't in control of the external circumstances that increase our stress levels. In many cases, getting pregnant and being pregnant are stressful enough on their own, notwithstanding life's other challenges.

In this chapter, we explain why reducing stress is so important for fertility and for having the best pregnancy possible. We'll also describe techniques you can use to reduce stress and give you tips for creating a low-stress environment.

Stress and Fertility

When a woman is stressed, her cortisol level rises. Cortisol is essential for life, but a chronic high level is damaging to health. A high cortisol level is bad for fertility because the body makes cortisol from progesterone. When your cortisol level rises, your progesterone level can fall, because the progesterone is used up. A shortage of progesterone can disrupt hormonal communication, leading to an irregular menstrual cycle and inhibited egg maturation. Furthermore, cortisol competes with progesterone for the same receptors (the cellular proteins that bind the hormone to make the cells work) in your body and your baby's body. If the body's progesterone is used up to make cortisol, a fertilized egg can't be maintained in the womb. Progesterone deficiency can also result in estrogen dominance, which is a common cause of premenstrual syndrome.

During pregnancy, higher cortisol and decreased progesterone discourages the growth signals that shape the intelligence and the sex of your baby. T. S. Wiley, an expert in bioidentical hormone replacement and the author of *Sex, Lies, and Menopause: The Shocking Truth about Synthetic Hormones and the Benefits of Natural Alternatives*, told us recently, "High levels of cortisol in Mom during pregnancy result in lifetime stress for the child." This is one of the reasons to consider a bioidentical progesterone cream before and during pregnancy.

Progesterone is documented to be a respiratory stimulant and to increase the oxygen level in the blood. In fact, largely as a result of progesterone, a woman's lung capacity increases by about 20 percent by the time her baby is born. We think that using bioidentical progesterone during pregnancy is safe and beneficial, as we discussed in chapter 8.

There are also nerve fibers that directly connect the brain to the ovaries. When a woman is under stress, these nerves can cause spasms in the fallopian tubes and uterus, possibly interfering with a fertilized egg. Consistent with these ideas, studies suggest that women conceive in the months when they are less stressed. For many couples, infertility itself is a source of stress.

Stress and Pregnancy

Stress hormones have both a protective and a damaging effect on the body. Many of them operate by boosting activity temporarily, forcing the body to work faster and harder at whatever it's doing. This provides for a faster response time and a greater ability to fight or flee from a threat. Given our dangerous environment, these hormones promote survival, but only when they act for short periods. The energy that goes into heightening response time always comes at a cost. If stress hormones are chronically elevated, disease accelerates and health begins to deteriorate. Experienced athletes who train for hours every day are among those with the highest risk of getting a disease. When exercised too much, the body extends beyond growth mode and enters a protective stress mode.

Stress harms an unborn baby for two main reasons. First, when the mother is under stress, her body works faster and becomes more vigilant. Naturally, this uses up more energy and resources. In the case of chronic stress, this means her body might be using energy and resources that her baby needs more than she does. But since the mother is stressed, her body doesn't know that and keeps the resources for itself.

Second, the mother's stress hormones send messages not just to her own cells but to her baby's. They prompt a protective fight-or-flight response in your baby even if that response isn't really necessary. A baby who senses stress in the womb starts using energy and resources faster, too, and also starts preparing for a life of stress outside the womb, even if life outside the womb isn't stressful at all.

There's a lot of research backing this up, especially regarding the development of your baby's brain. When the mother is stressed, her higher cortisol and other stress-hormone levels signal her baby that it's not safe to continue in full growth mode. When her baby enters defense mode, the growth of neurons and synapses in the brain is slowed or inhibited. Sometimes the production of fewer nerve receptors causes a physical reprogramming of the brain, making way for the baby to have a lifelong tendency to become stressed easily.

A study of 156 unborn children measured the effect of maternal stress by drawing blood samples from pregnant women and asking them to fill out questionnaires on their emotional states. Once that was completed, the researchers mildly stimulated the unborn child through the mother's abdomen and measured fetal heart rate. The babies of the stressed mothers responded more quickly, sustaining faster heartbeats for longer periods. The babies of the mothers reporting the lowest stress levels had heartbeats that returned to normal most quickly. (Higher fetal heart rate has been linked to heart disease and diabetes later in life.) Mothers who experienced depression during pregnancy tended to have babies who cried more and were difficult to soothe.

High stress in a pregnant woman can even lead to disorders like ADHD and autism in genetically susceptible babies. Much research backs this up. Babies born to mothers under stress while pregnant were found to have a higher rate of motor problems and ADHD. Children who were exposed to excessive maternal stress in the womb showed a greater tendency for anxiety and depression later in life. Mothers of schizophrenics were almost two times as likely to have rated themselves as depressed during the sixth or seventh month of pregnancy. Mothers with emotional difficulties had babies who had higher rates of sleep disorders, digestive problems, and irritability.

All of this makes perfect sense, given our newfound knowledge of epigenetics—it's due to premature defensive (as opposed to growth) brain patterns that the fetus develops in response to high levels of stress hormones like adrenaline and cortisol. Conversely, a low-stress, peaceful, and happy womb environment is accompanied by feel-good endorphins and hormones like oxytocin that promote a sense of well-being in your baby. This allows for optimal brain development and stays with him or her for life.

In extreme cases, chronic high stress can effect the outcome of a pregnancy. Women who reported high levels of anxiety and stress have been found to give birth at an earlier gestational stage and to babies with lower birth weight. The more anxiety and stress a woman described, the lower the weight of her baby was. A group of Michigan researchers found that unmarried women or women in low-income families were more likely to miscarry. Extremely stressed women, such as women who experience domestic abuse during pregnancy, are also more prone to use normal street drugs like tobacco and alcohol to deal with the stress.

When these substances are coupled with the mother's stress hormones, the baby often can't survive the environment. Women in these situations are at high risk of premature birth, low–birth weight babies, miscarriage, or stillbirth. These situations usually aren't the mother's fault at all.

Where Does Stress Come From?

A variety of circumstances can lead to stress. It usually takes a combination of them in succession to create chronic high stress. But knowing what's causing your stress can sometimes help you to deal with it and release the emotions. Common sources of stress include the following:

- Unhealthy diet
- Toxins in the body
- Family, relationship, or marital problems
- Financial hardship
- Legal conflict
- Grief or loss of a loved one
- Trouble with communication
- Pressure to perform at work or school
- Addiction
- Health issues
- Time management and scheduling
- Adaptation to change
- Anger issues
- Travel or large life adjustment (good or bad)
- Difficult daily routine (like heavy traffic)
- Unrealistic expectations
- Fear and uncertainty about being pregnant
- Sleep quality issues

Keeping maternal stress low isn't entirely a mother's responsibility. Her husband or partner has an enormous supporting role to play in keeping her peaceful, calm, happy, and stress-free. Before getting pregnant, a couple can reduce stress by cultivating a harmonious, interdependent relationship that supports the woman emotionally and minimizes her stress level. Of course, if the man works to reduce his own stress level, it keeps stress low for his partner, too. We also have a hunch that while a couple is trying to conceive, lower stress in the man leads to better sperm quality.

Aside from outward behavior, internal health issues involving the endocrine system can effect the signals your baby receives. We recommend consulting with a holistic or antiaging physician and taking comprehensive adrenal stress, thyroid, and hormone tests before getting pregnant. Our diet, detox, and stress-reducing methods will help in all categories, but it's important to find out where you stand. Short bursts of stress are natural and aren't very harmful to your baby. It's chronic, ongoing stress that distracts your unborn baby from growing, keeping him or her in a costly protection mode.

What to Do about Stress

Our entire program reduces stress. Eating the right foods gives the body the fuel it needs to handle stress. Toxins and unhealthy foods are themselves a source of stress. That's one reason we eliminate them in our program. Getting enough sleep gives the body time to regenerate, and techniques like exercise, yoga, mindful breathing, meditation, and heart rate variability training reduce the body's stress response. We cover these techniques next and then get into other factors that affect your stress level, like jaw tension, thyroid health, infectious disease, travel, and even the type of lighting in your home or office.

In addition to using these techniques, a simple way to reduce stress is to ask for help when you need it. Support from family, friends, counselors, community agencies, and religious advisers can go a long way in restoring a mother to health and a baby to growth. It's well-known that if a woman shares her emotional baggage, frustrations, and other sources of stress or depression with someone who cares, her burden is lightened. If she finds herself even a little stressed, talking about it with a loved one or getting support will do more than she realizes for her baby. She needs emotional support more during pregnancy than at any other time of life, because this is when her stress-hormone levels can affect her baby's growth profoundly, especially brain development. And, as usual, this advice is not just for women—men would do well to share, too.

No matter what happens, reducing stress can be as simple as doing your best at everything and knowing you did. After all, that's all we can do. When people are content with their situations in life, stress is naturally lower. But stress is increased dramatically when the current situation isn't what we want it to be. Sometimes this is health related and can be corrected by rebalancing brain chemicals, but at other times a change in one's outlook on life is what's needed. Thanks to breakthrough science in psychology and physiology, now more than ever we have access to resources that can help us to improve our attitudes and find contentment and happiness in life.

Sleep

Sleep is your body's time to rest, heal, and regenerate. Getting enough sleep is central to fertility and to a healthy pregnancy and baby. In the 1960s, it was average for Americans to report getting eight to nine hours of sleep every night. Now they report getting only seven. Six to nine hours of sleep a night is sufficient for most adults, although individuals do have various needs and may require more or (in rare cases) less. Pregnant women usually need more, especially during the first trimester.

Proper hormone (endocrine system) function is heavily dependent on a quality sleep cycle. This includes metabolism in particular. The pituitary gland, the master endocrine gland that controls the release of hormones from other glands, is sensitive to sleep loss. The root of this process lies in the pineal gland, a tiny endocrine gland in the center of the brain. The pineal gland is made of nerve and retinal tissues. It is light-sensitive and serves as your biological clock, regulating the circadian rhythm (the twenty-four-hour cycle), including sleep and wakefulness, with hormones like melatonin and cortisol.

The circadian rhythm is the scheduled biochemical, physiological, and behavioral changes that living organisms go through every day. Your body establishes its circadian rhythm in response to the levels of certain types of light, being especially sensitive to the presence and absence of sunlight. Your body resists resetting your circadian rhythm. This means that the sun rising and setting each day actually has an extreme influence on your body's activities.

In order to stimulate the release of sex hormones, the hypothalamus relies on receiving certain messages from the pineal gland through the pituitary gland, making the reproductive cycle heavily dependent on healthy, regular pineal activity. And to have healthy, regular pineal activity, you have to get plenty of regular sleep.

If the sleep pattern is disrupted, pineal activity is disrupted. Sleep-pattern disruption can occur from insomnia, poor lighting conditions in the bedroom, stress, and travel involving a time-zone shift (jet lag). When pineal activity is disrupted, the hypothalamus-pituitary axis is disrupted, and the menstrual cycle and sperm production are impaired. Appetite control and insulin metabolism are also affected, making sleep deprivation a factor in diabetes and obesity. As little as one hour of sleep disruption over the course of several days is enough to decrease cognitive function. If sleep deprivation continues for a longer period, depression can result. A study of women in professions that require frequent partial sleep deprivation found that a staggering 50 percent reported irregular menstrual cycles. Compare that to 20 percent for the general female population.

If you don't feel rested during daylight hours without the use of artificial stimulants like caffeine, try getting more regular sleep. A good gauge of this is to see how you feel right after you wake up, not after you've been up for a while. If you still feel groggy, go back to sleep. If you can't because you have to get up for work, that means your body needs you to go to bed a little earlier the next night.

It's important to sleep in a room that is pitch-black (no light at all from any source). This not only means no TV, computer, or smartphone screens, it also means no hall light shining through a slightly open door, no street light shining through a window, no digital clock—nothing. The light receptors in your eyes are very sensitive, and seeing even the smallest amount of light can keep your pineal gland on a wakefulness program, which inevitably affects sex-hormone levels. You may not even notice a light level that can affect this.

Women sleeping in lighted quarters have more patchy mucus, short luteal phases (the days after ovulation and before menstruation), and other menstrual irregularities. These irregularities often cause infertility. Irregular, infertile women have become regular in one to three cycles and pregnant in about five cycles simply by removing all light from their sleeping quarters. Light in sleeping quarters has also been associated with early-term miscarriage. Going to bed at exactly the same time isn't nearly as important as providing your body with sufficient time for sleep in total darkness.

Here are a few tips for getting healthy sleep:

- Don't eat snacks right before bed, especially if they're high in sugar or carbohydrates. High blood sugar inhibits healthy sleep. Small amounts of raw honey are okay.

- Within an hour before going to sleep, stop looking at screens, including cell phones, computers, and televisions. These units provide a great deal of stimulation to the brain and can keep you awake longer than you want. If it's necessary to use a computer, there is software that can modify your operating system to decrease screen brightness and optimize hues to decrease eyestrain.

- Try to get to bed by 11:00 p.m. Your body tries to do most of its regeneration between 11:00 p.m. and 1:00 a.m., and this regeneration won't really happen if you're awake—at least not as much.

- Don't keep your room too hot.

- Don't sleep on a bed with metal in it. For a detailed explanation of this, see chapter 10.

- If you really can't get your room pitch-black, wear a black eye mask.

- If giving your body eight to nine hours of darkness doesn't keep you alert, wakeful, and clear-minded throughout the next day, there's a deeper issue at hand. Possible culprits include caffeine addiction, chronic fatigue, toxicity, nutritional deficiency, or poor sleep quality from a condition like sleep apnea. If getting more sleep in total darkness doesn't help, we recommend seeing a holistic physician. Remember how harmful high levels of stress hormones are for your baby? Stress-hormone levels rise especially when you're short on proper sleep. If you aren't sleeping well, correcting this before pregnancy will be a big help to your baby.

Exercise

Getting in shape during the six months before pregnancy is helpful because most beneficial types of exercise become difficult as pregnancy progresses. Being in shape before you get pregnant gives you a huge advantage during the pregnancy and especially during the recovery period after giving birth.

By "in shape," we certainly don't mean preparing for a marathon. Like most things, exercise is best done moderately. Two to three times a week of vigorous exercise (in which you reach the point of not being able to continue) is usually about right. Although a sedentary lifestyle isn't healthy, four hours of hard exercise every day isn't healthy, either.

Exercise burns energy, but it actually keeps your energy level high.

Exercise strengthens the heart, lungs, and muscles. Muscles are meant to be used. Inactivity deprives the muscles of the nutrients they need to stay healthy and inhibits their ability to respond to insulin and absorb blood sugar for energy use. That leads to too much insulin in the bloodstream, which promotes obesity and endangers ovulation, conception, and pregnancy. Aside from not eating sugar, physical activity is the best way to keep blood sugar and insulin in check. Exercise helps people to lose weight not because it burns energy but primarily because it increases insulin sensitivity and lowers the insulin level. A high insulin level signals the body to store fat for later use. Exercise is essential for women who are having trouble getting pregnant because of an insulin issue.

Our bodies weaken and waste away if we don't use them. In 1966, a study was conducted in which five healthy men spent three weeks of their summer vacations in bed. Before their time in bed, the men weren't lazy, depressed, or fatigued, and they had no major health issues. When the men got out of bed three weeks later, they had a higher heart rate, a weaker heart, higher blood pressure, more body fat, and less lean muscle than before.

After that the men started on an eight-week exercise program designed to reverse the deterioration caused by the excessive bed rest. By the end of the eight weeks, some of the men were in better shape than they had been before the study. Thirty years later, the researchers found the same five men and discovered that they had gained an average of fifty pounds and had lower heart strength. They started a six-month walking, jogging, and cycling program, after which their heart rates, blood pressure, and maximum heart-pumping power returned to the same values they had been before the initial study began thirty years earlier.

Researchers conducted a similar bed-rest study of older men and women of average age sixty-seven. The older people lost more muscle in ten days than the young men in the earlier study had lost in a month. The older you get, the more important it is to use your body. Getting good exercise is one of the best ways to prevent common diseases.

Yet even though it's critical to get good exercise, too much causes excess cortisol release and puts the body under stress. It's also important not to be too lean—you definitely want to have some fat reserves. In the 1970s, Rose E. Frisch, an associate professor of population sciences at Harvard, observed women who worked diligently to keep their weight low, like gymnasts, swimmers, and marathon runners. She noticed that these women often stopped having monthly periods during intense exercise. A day or two of rest each week was enough to boost their fat levels enough to jump-start regular menstruation. A small amount of fat storage is healthy and even necessary for normal bodily function. Women who had regular menstrual cycles were then asked to engage in intense exercise for several weeks to see if the reverse effect occurred, and indeed it did. The intense exercise caused irregular menstruation in women who had been regular before the exercise.

The combination of heavy exercise and decreased fat reserves interferes with the hypothalamus's ability to generate gonadotropin-releasing hormone. Without this hormone, the pituitary gland isn't signaled to produce enough luteinizing hormone, which is required to cause eggs to mature and be released from the ovaries. This disrupts ovulation and shuts down the menstrual cycle. From the standpoint of survival, this makes perfect sense: the woman's body knows that it doesn't have enough stored energy to conduct a successful pregnancy. So even though some exercise is important to keep the insulin level low enough to become pregnant, exercising too much will actually shut down the female reproductive cycle. If you are exercising daily, you may want to reduce the frequency of your workouts, or at least increase the amount of sweet potatoes or rice you eat for dinner on workout days.

Types of Exercise

Exercise falls into two main categories: aerobic and resistance. Aerobic exercise is any continuous activity that uses up oxygen in the blood by working most of the body, causing the breathing and heart rates to increase. Swimming, running, walking, and cycling are examples of aerobic exercise. Resistance exercise usually works specific muscle groups. Your heart rate will go up during resistance exercise, but not as much as during aerobic exercise. Weight lifting, push-ups, pull-ups, sit-ups, and the like are all resistance exercises. They strengthen the muscles and promote a lean body mass. Both types of exercise increase insulin sensitivity.

Aerobic exercise requires more oxygen. It increases heart strength, basal metabolic rate, and pulse pressure and decreases resting heart rate, blood pressure, and body fat percentage. Oxygen delivery to the tissues is improved dramatically with regular aerobic exercise, which makes the body function better at every task. Resistance exercise similarly increases basal metabolic rate. Resistance exercise causes faster excess weight loss and improves the body's fat profile. Although aerobic and resistance exercise offer different benefits, one isn't better than the other. A good exercise program includes both.

Why Exercise Is So Important for Fertility

The most important thing about exercise for fertility and pregnancy is that it increases insulin sensitivity. A study of twenty-six thousand women found that fertility was directly correlated with exercise. This is true because too much insulin promotes infertility. Insulin regulates the blood sugar level by escorting excess sugar into the body tissues, primarily the fat cells. Insulin is chemically similar to ovarian hormones that regulate the female reproductive cycle and help eggs to mature.

When the insulin level is elevated for an extended period, insulin blocks the receptors on the ovaries that are intended to receive ovarian hormones. Insulin does not promote egg maturity when attached to these receptors, so egg maturity will be delayed as long as insulin is occupying the receptors. The ovaries confuse the attached insulin with their own growth factors and actually decrease the production of their own hormones.

When excess insulin is attached to the receptors, it also stimulates the ovaries to produce excess androgen, disrupting the hormonal balance. Harmful consequences of excess androgen include cosmetic issues like acne, excess body hair, and changes in the blood lipid profile associated with heart disease. Insulin also blocks the enzymes that rupture the follicle wall at the time of ovulation. The overall effect of eating lots of sugar is progression toward infertility and illness.

Exercise (and eating a low-sugar diet) keeps the insulin level low by burning glucose instead of sending it back to the bloodstream. Regular use of muscle tissue improves the functioning of the mitochondria, the power plants inside cells that convert nutrients into energy. When you don't exercise, the mitochondria slow down. This is important in insulin sensitivity, because glucose isn't able to get into skeletal muscle tissue on its own—it requires a special protein called GLUT4.

GLUT4 picks up glucose from the blood and carries it through the cell membranes and into the muscle cells, where the glucose is used as fuel. If mitochondrial function is poor, free fatty acids running through the blood build up around the muscle cells and make it difficult or impossible for GLUT4 to get into them. Properly functioning mitochondria are able to clear away the free fatty acids and allow GLUT4 to do its job. When GLUT4 is refused, glucose remains in the blood and the insulin level rises.

If this situation is ongoing, insulin resistance will develop as more and more insulin is needed to regulate the blood sugar. People who have developed insulin resistance have up to 30 percent less mitochondria than people who don't have insulin resistance. This is usually the direct result of a lack of exercise. Physical inactivity results in a fast decline in oxygen uptake and mitochondrial activity. Aerobic exercise is the best way to oxygenate the body. It increases the overall mitochondrial surface area, which boosts mitochondrial function and increases insulin sensitivity. As your body gains a better ability to use oxygen, it becomes stronger and endurance increases. Short bursts of intense aerobic and resistance exercise together increase insulin sensitivity the most.

Exercise also causes the body to use energy. The body's storage unit for excess energy is adipose tissue, commonly called body fat. Adipose tissue is not a passive storage location; it's live tissue that sends signals to the rest of the body by producing hormones that influence appetite, the desire for physical activity, weight, and the reproductive cycle. Adiponectin is a common protein made by adipose tissue that triggers the fat-burning processes, making the cells more sensitive to insulin and enhancing ovulation.

The more weight a person gains, however, the less adiponectin the adipose tissue is able to make. A lower level of adiponectin promotes insulin resistance. Extra body fat also boosts interleukin-6, which interferes with the ability of a fertilized egg to implant itself in the uterine lining. If a woman is ten pounds overweight, it's not an issue, but if she's obese, there's a chance it's interfering with her hormone levels and contributing to infertility.

Yoga: Aerobic and Resistance Exercise All in One

Originating in India several thousand years ago, yoga is a system of postures and movements that combines aerobic and resistance exercises. The purpose of yoga is to heal the body while rejuvenating and sharpening the mind and the spirit, helping you to reach a stress-free state of contentment.

Yoga postures and movements strengthen the physical body and increase flexibility, both of which help throughout pregnancy, especially the third trimester. These postures and movements are often far outside our normal range of motion. Many people who practice yoga for the first time say that they feel muscles in their bodies that they didn't know existed. Through these postures and movements, yoga increases the blood flow and carries healing, detoxifying oxygen to deeper places in the body. It also corrects imbalances in muscle tightness that can promote stress. When these imbalances are removed, people feel more in tune with their bodies.

Imbalances can come from physical activity (or lack thereof) or negative emotions. Negative emotions like anger, fear, and resentment have noticeably damaging effects on health, and they're dangerous for a fetus. Yoga heals the body from the effects of these emotions and promotes clean energy flow throughout the body.

When combined with breathing exercises and meditation, yoga detoxifies the body and stimulates the endocrine system. It also promotes a greater awareness of one's body. A tangible objective in yoga is to become calm enough to sit with a quiet mind (that is, meditate). When this becomes refreshing, yoga is starting to work.

We've already discussed the significant, lifelong effects that stress in a mother can have on a fetus. The powerful ability of yoga to reduce stress makes it our exercise of choice for having a healthy baby. Yoga reduces stress by increasing our awareness of the ways in which our bodies create and store stress and tension. When we become more aware of stress and stress patterns, we're better able to identify the sources of our stress. Once you know what's causing your stress, you can remove the conditions or change the behavior.

Prenatal yoga classes have the added benefit of giving you a social network of other expectant mothers. It's okay if you've never done yoga before. All yoga studios offer beginners' classes, and most provide mats for you, too. All you have to do is wear loose or stretchy workout clothes, show up, and do what the teacher says. You're better off at a dedicated yoga studio than at a health club or gym that also offers yoga. The classes are smaller at studios, and the teachers are usually better, so you'll get more and better attention.

There are many forms of yoga; we encourage you to try several until you find one you like. Yoga videos are fine once you've learned how to do the postures, but you'll need a teacher in a yoga studio for the first few months, at least. The following types of yoga are the most common:

- *Iyengar*. A traditional form that focuses on precisely aligned postures.

- *Ashtanga.* A traditional form that focuses on an ordered series of postures. It's important to have a good instructor so you learn the postures without hurting yourself. This is best tried before pregnancy.

- *Anusara.* A newer form that focuses on alignment, fun, and opening the heart. This is our favorite form of yoga.

- *Vinyasa.* A form in which you flow from one posture to another.

- *Bikram.* A form completed in a saunalike heated room. It's great for detoxing, but you should not attend a class if you are pregnant or think you might be. It's too hot.

Doing yoga two or three times a week will completely transform your body, and we think it fully satisfies the exercise part of our program. This goes for men, too. It's not unpleasant to go to yoga and see your significant other dressed in tight, stretchy clothing, flexing his or her muscles!

T-Tapp: Get the Most Exercise in the Least Amount of Time

If you're short on time, the absolutely best way to pack the most exercise into the least amount of time is Teresa Tapp's program, Fit and Fabulous in Fifteen Minutes. Tapp is a renowned fitness expert and exercise physiologist in Florida who has designed many of her own workouts and has worked with professional fashion models. Her program is known, for short, as "T-Tapp."

T-Tapp workouts are short, less than twenty minutes each. They are a variety of very specifically designed movements you perform without weights, sort of like an aerobics class. The difference here is that the goal is not aerobic training but muscle fitness and circulation and excretion of toxins in the body.

The T-Tapp workout we like best is called the Basic Plus Workout. It takes just fifteen minutes and covers all of the basics of exercise in just the right amounts. Like many forms of yoga, T-Tapp has the following outstanding effects:

- Detoxifying the body
- Increasing insulin sensitivity

- Reducing stress
- Increasing energy level and mental clarity
- Boosting metabolism
- Improving cardiovascular function
- Helping the brain to gain better control over the body (building the neurokinetic function)

T-Tapp Basic Plus is the premier preconception detox workout, because so many of the movements are designed to maximize lymphatic circulation. The lymphatic system is one of the body's primary ways of eliminating toxins. There are lymph nodes and pathways that appear much like blood vessels and run throughout your body, which uses them as channels for eliminating toxins. The lymphatic system is not pumped by the heart, however; it's pumped when we move. That's why T-Tapp is so effective at detoxing.

T-Tapp is one of our favorites in terms of consistency because you don't have to drive anywhere and it takes just fifteen minutes; it's so convenient that it's easy to stick with it. T-Tapp will also dramatically improve your physique. Dave was the first one of us to try T-Tapp, while he was in a hotel room on a business trip for several days. When he got back, Lana noticed he had developed tighter abdominal muscles and wondered what he'd been doing. Soon she started it for herself. You truly will see the effects within days. We highly recommend doing T-Tapp if you're short on time, on days you don't make it to yoga, or if you're just not a yoga fan. We include links to our favorite workouts on www.betterbabybook.com/exercise.

Other Exercise Options

If none of our suggestions thus far appeal to you, here are a few principles to consider when designing your own exercise program. You'll probably see the best results by focusing on resistance exercises. This is exactly what yoga and T-Tapp do.

For aerobics, low-impact exercises like swimming or riding a bicycle are the healthiest. Jogging on pavement or even on a treadmill is hard on the body, especially the joints. Soon after you're pregnant, your body will produce a hormone called relaxin that makes your ligaments stretchy, which is not always comfortable if your joints are accustomed to being pounded on pavement. Walking at a fast pace is better for you than jogging, whether you're on a treadmill, the pavement, or grass. If you have trouble getting a vigorous aerobic workout from walking alone, try increasing the incline of the treadmill. If you're walking up a ten- to fifteen-degree incline, you can get an excellent low-impact workout just by walking quickly. Do not do this in the third trimester, however, because your ligaments become so loose in preparation for birth that this type of exercise can cause your lower back to become less stable.

Lifting light weights once or twice a week is a good resistance routine. Our experience is that most forms of yoga are incredible muscle workouts. Dave stopped lifting weights entirely in favor of doing yoga and actually increased his muscle mass.

Whether you choose weightlifting or yoga, exercising to the point of not being able to continue gives you the best workout. Weight-bearing exercise makes your bones stronger, and it will make your growth hormone spike if you eat protein within fifteen minutes of finishing your workout. A spike in growth hormone can help you get pregnant because it rejuvenates your entire system.

Overexercising

Earlier we mentioned that exercising too much can promote infertility. This is because overexercising increases the stress level throughout the body, which can disrupt a woman's menstrual cycle. Low-stress exercises like yoga or T-Tapp are our top choices, because they combine powerful stress-reducing effects: exercise, deep breathing, detoxification, and meditation. Reducing stress promotes fertility in men and women and creates an environment in a woman's body that welcomes her new baby.

If you're doing regular workouts, we recommend forty-five-minute-or-less workouts only two or three times a week before pregnancy. If you want to exercise every day, you can do the T-Tapp Basic Plus Workout or go for a light walk on the days you're not doing cardio or yoga.

During pregnancy, prenatal yoga and low-stress exercises like cycling, Pilates, swimming, and walking are best. Many women have also done T-Tapp throughout their pregnancies with great success. After the fourth month of pregnancy, avoid exercising while lying on your back. The expanding uterus can compress the vena cava, the main vein that carries blood back to the heart. Lying on your back will increase the chance of this compression. Also avoid exercises that require holding your breath, because maintaining your baby's oxygen supply at this time is critical. Finally, avoid prolonged or overheated exercise. An unborn baby thrives only when its mother's body temperature is below 102.5 degrees Fahrenheit.

What Exercise Does for Your Baby

When you exercise the right way, it benefits your baby. The American Physiological Society reports that safe exercise during pregnancy helps a fetus's nervous system to develop. The study demonstrated that the fetuses of exercising mothers had better control during breathing movements than the fetuses of nonexercising mothers. Also, just like their exercising mothers, the fetuses had lower average heart rates than the fetuses of the sedentary mothers.

When to Avoid Exercise

If you have any of the following conditions, you should avoid exercise during pregnancy:

- Intrauterine growth retardation
- Pregnancy-induced high blood pressure, uncontrolled blood pressure, a systolic (top number) over 160, or a diastolic (bottom number) over 100
- Premature rupture of membranes or placenta previa (in which the placenta blocks the opening from the uterus to the cervix)
- Persistent bleeding during the second and third trimester
- Preterm labor, in either the current pregnancy or a previous one
- Incompetent cervix (in which the fetus may spontaneously abort) and cerclage (a surgical procedure to close the cervix and keep the fetus intact in the uterus)
- A history of chronic high blood pressure, overactive thyroid, cardiovascular pulmonary disease, or miscarriage
- Multiple fetuses (twins, triplets, or more)

- Asthma
- Unstable angina

If you experience any of these situations, we recommend consulting with a holistic physician before beginning an exercise program.

Breathing Techniques (*Pranayama*)

Pranayama is a system of breathing used in many forms of yoga. The Sanskrit word *pranayama* means "breath control." Yogis (yoga masters) believe that breathing brings life energy (*prana*) into the body. They consider *prana* to be divine. *Prana* can also be taken into the body through natural foods and loving relationships.

Yogis believe that *prana* is drained from the body by stress, physical illness, prolonged strenuous exercise, an unhealthy diet, or a negative mindset. *Pranayama* is a powerful stress-reduction technique, because it increases and purifies our life energy and counteracts activities like stress that reduce *prana*.

Breathing itself is a highly unique bodily function, because it falls under both conscious control and unconscious control. For instance, you can think about breathing and breathe in certain ways, but if you stop thinking about breathing, your body will still do it for you. There's a deep mutual connection between the mind and breath control. The mind controls how we breathe, and our breathing affects how we think.

Consider how when you're upset you breathe faster, and when you're relaxed you breathe more slowly. Telling someone to "take a deep breath" when they're upset is good advice, because breathing more slowly really does serve to calm you down. The physical benefits of *pranayama* are extensive, and they include reduced cortisol level, decreased heart rate, and increased blood flow. *Pranayama* techniques are very powerful; no matter what you believe about *prana* and divine energy, we know you'll feel a big difference if you practice it every day.

We think it's important to take classes from a trained teacher or a yogi on a regular basis. Breathing in this conscious manner for at least ten minutes a day helps tremendously. If you don't practice this breathing technique every day, *pranayama* won't be nearly as effective when you get into a stressful situation and really need it.

Breathing techniques like *pranayama* have been shown to noticeably improve the quality of life for asthma patients. In addition, the Art of Living Foundation of Bangalore, India, which teaches breathing exercises in 152 countries, has taught breathing exercises in a number of U.S. prisons. In the prisons where it was taught, a 38 percent decrease in fighting was reported.

Meditation

Meditation is simply becoming more aware of your thoughts and feelings. When a thought comes up, instead of engaging it emotionally or intellectually or judging it, you acknowledge it and send it on its way, emptying your mind until the next thought surfaces. In a sense, you act as a third-party observer of your own thoughts. Sometimes further thoughts won't surface, and you'll be able to maintain a calm consciousness free of interruption for as long as you like. With practice, it becomes easier to reach and maintain this quiet state.

The positive health effects of meditation have been well documented for more than fifty years. Meditation lowers heart rate, blood pressure, body temperature, and cortisol level. It promotes the release of thyroid-stimulating hormone and human growth hormone and increases L-arginine and vasopressin levels. Arginine and vasopressin help with memory and learning. Meditation also reduces stress and fear and promotes clarity of mind.

Herbert Benson of Harvard Medical School is the founder and president of the Mind/Body Medical Institute. He found that Americans who practice meditation have lower oxygen metabolism (that is, they require less oxygen for healing and stress responses). Dr. Benson conducted a study of ninety patients with chronic pain. When the patients were put on a ten-week meditation program, they showed significant reductions in pain, negative body image, anxiety, and depression. Their use of drugs for pain management declined after the program, and most of the ninety patients continued meditating on their own.

Heart Rate Variability Training

Since the early 1990s, researchers at the Institute of HeartMath in Boulder Creek, California, have studied the relationship between the heart and the brain. Their findings are nothing short of astounding. They found that the heart actually has its own independent nervous system that makes decisions separately from the brain. Of all the nerves that run between the heart and the brain, 80 percent carry information from the heart to the brain, and only 20 percent carry information from the brain to the heart.

Our emotional states are reflected in our heart rhythms. Since the heart is the strongest source of rhythmic physical vibrations in the human body, the rest of the body's systems align with the heartbeat. If your emotional state is one of stress, your entire body feels the effects. The influence goes both ways: the heart profoundly influences the brain's emotional center (the amygdala), too. When the heart and the brain align in purpose instead of fighting for control, this heightens mental clarity, intelligence, and intuition. When the desires of the heart and the brain conflict, the brain and the heart fight for control and create incoherence throughout the body, raising a person's stress level.

Core heart feelings like love and compassion reduce the activity of the sympathetic nervous system (which facilitates stress responses) and increase the activity of the parasympathetic nervous system (which calms us from stress). Positive emotions like appreciation, care, compassion, happiness, and love improve hormonal balance and strengthen the immune system. People used to think that a steady heartbeat was healthy, but now we know that a heart in high coherence—that is, aligned in purpose with the brain—speeds up and slows down in a steady pattern that resembles a sine wave.

Coherence is exactly what we want for a mother during pregnancy to keep her fetus in growth mode. The researchers at HeartMath discovered that we can use our hearts and brains together to activate these positive emotions, purposefully creating a state of head-heart coherence. Now you can buy a simple device based on the HeartMath emWave technology that tells you when you're in coherence and confirms that your stress levels are falling. It's the fastest and easiest way we know to reduce stress and to know that you've reduced your stress.

Practicing coherence with emWave technology takes just a few minutes a day. Research has shown that when you practice coherence over time, your coherence baseline actually increases, meaning that you're naturally in coherence more of the day than you were before. For more information, visit www.betterbabybook.com/heartmath. This is the single best stress reducer we know, and Dave is a certified heart math coach and consultant.

Dealing with Travel

Even if you don't feel it much, travel substantially increases your stress level. Jet travel across time zones can disrupt the body's circadian rhythm and routine. When presented with a new time zone, a new light-dark cycle, and a new temperature, your body needs to adapt, but it resists these changes.

The process of adapting to a new environment is stressful for the body. And if it's stressful for a mother, it's stressful for her unborn baby. Hormone excretion cycles and body temperature have to catch up to the new schedule, and most of the time this is accompanied by sleep deprivation because of the travel experience. For a woman to be fertile and experience a regular menstrual cycle, maintaining a regular sleep-wake schedule is essential. Since travel often disrupts this, we suggest minimizing travel before and during pregnancy if you can.

These days, traveling exposes us to lots of toxins, too. Airplane cabins contain more than 80 percent recirculated air. Pilots allegedly get as much as ten times more oxygen than passengers do. This low oxygen environment is bad for fertility and especially harmful for a fetus. General travel stress also leads to elevated adrenaline and cortisol levels. The close proximity to many people, the reduced oxygen level in the body, and the recirculation of air raise the risk of contracting infectious diseases, particularly upper respiratory ones. They are transmitted when an infected person sneezes and coughs or touches surfaces such as door knobs. With the air being 80 percent recirculated, you don't even have to be sitting near someone to be exposed to these pathogens.

Airlines frequently reduce the air circulation level in the cabin to reduce the flight cost. Fainting, nausea, and headaches among passengers happen sometimes because of the lack of oxygen. Getting an asthma oxygen inhaler from your doctor to use on a flight can help. If you fly, wearing a surgical mask can reduce your exposure to contaminated air. Of course, most air travelers don't wear surgical masks, but we've seen plenty of people wear them, so you might not be the only one doing so. You can also drizzle drinking water on a handkerchief or surgical mask to humidify your own air supply and alleviate dizziness, light-headedness, and goofy feelings. We wouldn't worry about this for a short flight.

On international flights, in order to prevent international transmission of crop-ruining insects, highly toxic pesticides may be sprayed directly into the air that passengers breathe, and mists settle on the skin. Planes heading into Australia, the Czech Republic, China, Cuba, Egypt, Grenada, India, Kenya, Kiribati, Madagascar, Nigeria, Senegal, the Seychelles, South Africa, Switzerland, Tahiti, Trinidad, Tobago, the United Kingdom, and Uruguay are sprayed. Planes to Barbados, the Cook Islands, Fiji, Jamaica, New Zealand, and Panama are sometimes treated with residual insecticides, which could easily harm passengers who board the planes later. If you fly to one of these countries during pregnancy, covering yourself with a blanket during the spraying will help.

Addressing Jaw Tension

Jaw tension can raise your stress level. A poor bite, such as an overbite or when the top front four teeth collide with the bottom front teeth, raises the level of a neuropeptide called substance P throughout the body. A high level of substance P is correlated with many health problems, including autoimmune conditions, which can interfere with pregnancy or cause health problems in a baby. Substance P can cause hypercoagulation of the blood, which is already a problem for some pregnant women. Substance P also blocks progesterone from doing its job.

Dr. Dwight Jennings, a dentist in Alameda, California, is one of the world's top experts on the effects of jaw tension. After more than twenty years of practice and clinical experience, Dr. Jennings believes that if there's a bad bite alignment in a mother, it can harm her baby, because it influences inflammation throughout the mother's nervous system. He had one patient who couldn't get pregnant for years. When he corrected her bite with a bite guard and splint, she got pregnant just four months later. Many of his other patients had suffered from spontaneous miscarriages but were able to have successful pregnancies after he corrected their jaw misalignments.

If you have any jaw pain or tension, or if your top front teeth hit your bottom front teeth when you close your mouth, consider seeing a specialist in temporomandibular joint disorder (TMJ). Dentists and orthodontists who specialize in TMJ can provide a splint or do bite realignment work with braces or other methods. This can lower jaw tension and substance P levels, which will boost fertility and the health of mother and baby. If seeing a specialist isn't practical, an inexpensive nighttime bite guard from your local drugstore can help, too. A simple way to deal with substance P directly is to take cayenne pepper capsules with your meals. Capsaicin, the hot part of chili peppers, depletes the body's substance P supply.

Lighting

In our modern society, we're exposed to hours of unnatural light from various kinds of bulbs. Most bulbs emit light that's just fine for our health, but there are a couple of types to avoid. The first is fluorescent bulbs, whether it's daytime or nighttime. The second is blue- or green-spectrum light at night. Blue- or green-spectrum light isn't harmful in itself, but it can disturb sleep patterns at night.

Fluorescent Light

John Ott, a twentieth-century photographer and cinematographer, was one of the first to study the effects of light on humans and animals. His research revealed that fluorescent bulbs damage our health. Perhaps because of fluorescent bulbs' flickering and glare, unnatural light spectrum, and ultraviolet light emission, people exposed to fluorescent lights have complained of blurred vision, dizziness, eyestrain, fatigue, headaches, mood swings, nausea, and other problems.

Fluorescent lights are believed to deplete vitamins A, B, and possibly D in the body, and deficiency in these vitamins corresponds with the symptoms fluorescents cause. Low B levels can result in fatigue, for example. Fluorescent bulbs also emit certain types of radiation, including X-rays and microwaves, which may explain their association with cancer, autism, ADHD, birth defects, and Alzheimer's disease. Fluorescent bulbs include not just the traditional long tubes but also the new compact fluorescent bulbs. In 2012, Stony Brook University researchers published a report on the release of cancer-promoting ultraviolet light from fluorescent bulbs. If you're exposed to fluorescent lights, try keeping the lights off and see if you feel better. You can also try full-spectrum bulbs (which fit in many standard fluorescent fixtures) or NaturaLux filters, which balance colors, eliminate glare, and cut radiation (including ultraviolet radiation) from fluorescents.

Sometimes it's not possible to turn the lights off because you're working in a public area. In this case, wearing sunglasses, polarized lenses, or glasses with built in yoke prisms can filter the light and produce less environmental stress.

It's ideal to depend on sunlight as much as possible during the day. As incandescent bulbs are phased out over the next several years, industry is pushing for the use of compact fluorescents. But for the reasons discussed here, we recommend opting for halogen, LED, or xenon lighting with high-quality dimmer switches. Low-quality dimmer switches result in flickering and EMF emission. Dimmer switches are great, because dimming the lights at night prepares you for going to sleep. The lower-intensity light allows the pineal gland to begin producing melatonin.

White or Blue- or Green-Spectrum Light

Light color and light intensity heavily influence our hormones and sleep cycles, with blue- and green-spectrum lights having particularly strong waking effects. When blue- or green-spectrum light (emitted in sunlight and most white light) is seen by the eyes, the pineal gland reduces melatonin production.

Other light colors, including red and ultraviolet, can suppress melatonin production as well, but they usually have to be very bright. With blue and green light, though, just a little—such as a blue LED in your bedroom—will stimulate wakefulness. This is why the best alarm clocks are manufactured with red displays.

Women wake up several times a night during pregnancy to use the bathroom, and after birth it's common to awaken in the middle of the night to nurse. If white, blue- or green-spectrum light is seen during these times, it can be very difficult to fall back to sleep. Insomnia may result, and ongoing insomnia and disrupted sleep patterns will lead to exhaustion and poor health for mom and baby.

Fortunately, there are dim LED nightlights on the market that emit no blue- or green-spectrum light at all. After we replaced our incandescent nightlights with LED nightlights, Lana found it very easy to return to sleep after waking in the middle of the night. We also found blackout curtains that completely block light, which is helpful for naps and sleeping during the daytime. We include links to suppliers of nightlights that do not interfere with melatonin production at www.betterbabybook.com /lighting. These are extra helpful after your baby arrives too, because they help babies sleep better too.

16

Does Intention Matter?

Much of the content of this book is based on hard science. The concepts are often tangible and easy to measure. Hard science likes it that way, and as a Silicon Valley executive and a medical doctor, we are always delighted when we find hard scientific confirmation for something we think is true.

Yet in the process of becoming advanced yoga students and learning to meditate, we discovered that even things that are hard to measure can matter—an awful lot. There are even hard scientific studies showing that 70 percent of women who "had a feeling" about the sex of their babies were right. What's more, 100 percent of women who dreamed about their baby's sex were right.

We aren't psychics, and we don't have any other special abilities. We're level-headed, normal people with professional degrees and jobs. We mention these types of unquantifiable experiences because when we shared them with our friends, we got more than a few smiles and nods, and other mothers related similar experiences back to us. It's more common than we realize, and it's a normal part of many of our lives. Lana hears these things often in her fertility practice.

An astonishing book, *The Intention Experiment: Using Your Thoughts to Change Your Life and the World* by Lynne McTaggart, summarizes a large body of research on how our attitudes and intentions can shape our future reality. Some new breakthroughs in quantum physics are even starting to support the findings. Books like *The Secret* by Rhonda Byrne and movies like *What the Bleep Do We Know?* are commonplace. Bruce Lipton's *The Biology of Belief* is another example of this line of thinking. The jury is still out on whether mainstream science accepts these ideas. But from our personal experience, we're sold. We do believe that intention plays a role in how our lives turn out, including the health of our children and whether we have children at all. We firmly believe that our expectation that we could and would get pregnant played a role in our success.

We certainly don't mean to say that people who are having difficulty conceiving don't want it enough—there are plenty of biochemical and lifestyle reasons that can make things go wrong. Nonetheless, knowing with certainty that you want to get pregnant and having faith that you will can help a lot with getting pregnant and having a healthy pregnancy. We even found some research supporting the notion that children who are wanted while they are in the womb have significantly better psychological profiles later in life.

For a couple to have the healthiest, happiest children possible, it's essential that they *want* children. Wanting your baby can be important for fertility, and after conception it's critical for your baby's health and well-being. Both partners' desire or lack of desire to have a child has a tremendous impact on your baby's entire life. This factor has a strong influence even before conception. Long before your baby's brain forms or she becomes fully conscious, every individual cell in the embryo or fetus maintains an experience-based unconscious memory. When sex is accompanied by feelings of sensuality and love, the egg is more likely to receive the sperm willingly and happily. Egg and sperm and all the cells they produce then carry an unconscious "memory" of peace, love, and well-being instead of indifference, violence, or stress.

Studies of children born to mothers who didn't want them showed low average birth weights, high infant mortality rates, and poor health and development. Unwanted babies are twice as likely to die within a month of being born. In one Czech study, the researchers tracked 2,290 babies born between 1961 and 1963. The babies were born to women who were twice denied abortions during their pregnancy with the studied babies. In case after case, the unwanted children had more physical and emotional handicaps than usual. The handicaps became more significant and more noticeable the older the children got (and they were tracked well into adulthood).

Scientists at the University of Michigan's Institute for Social Research found in 1999 that unwanted children almost always have lower self-esteem than wanted children. Much of this is probably due to the mother's ongoing release of stress hormones. Since she doesn't want the baby, and the pregnancy itself is stressful for her, every time she looks at her body and is reminded of it, she's stressed instead of filled with joy.

To achieve the best health for their children, parents need to create a sense of calm and love from before conception onward. We think that maintaining this throughout pregnancy and your child's entire life has more benefits than scientists yet understand. And it will benefit you as much as it benefits your children. A child conceived and raised in love will benefit from that forever. Before we had our children, we both knew that we wanted them. If you don't really want children, the scientific evidence says that it's best not to have them, even if you're getting pressure from others.

17

The Best Way to Welcome Baby: A Gentle Birth

Whether you choose to have your baby at the hospital or at home, there are many things you can do to improve the experience for both mother and baby. Our recommendations in this chapter are designed to encourage your baby to stay in growth mode as much as possible through the birth process, transforming birth from a traumatic event to a comfortable time for the family with minimal stress. These things will make your baby's birth a gentle birth.

A Mother's Eyes

Right after giving birth, a mother is in a state of consciousness that's unlike any other. This state of consciousness usually follows immediately after the baby is born (that is, leaves the birth canal). There may be a brief period of involuntary uterine contractions during which a new mother can't engage in much physical voluntary movement. It is a way for the body to catch its "breath" after giving birth. Moments later, the new mother will look at her child and touch him and take him in her arms to initiate the first eye-to-eye contact. The baby's eyes are usually large and wide, due to the heightened level of norepinephrine released during birth.

This initial eye contact is an important part of early mother-baby interaction, and some research suggests it plays a significant role in a baby's development. Niko Tinbergen, who shared the 1973 Nobel Prize in physiology, studied autistic children by living with families who had an autistic child. He was convinced that a number of factors surrounding birth—like labor induction, anesthesia during labor, and delivery with forceps—may contribute to autism. He also believed that initial eye contact was a key factor for the baby's later social development.

Much of human interaction occurs with eye contact. Given that autistic children avoid eye contact with people, Tinbergen suspected that the disruption or prevention of eye contact between a mother and her baby right after birth might be a factor in autism. If a practice this simple might prevent autism, it is well worth the effort, although we are in no way convinced that autism is caused by, or even related to, eye contact. Regardless of its effect on health, the period of first eye contact is an extremely rewarding and special time for a new mother, and it certainly *feels* like something powerful and important is happening.

Self-Attachment

Self-attachment is the process by which a baby finds the mother's nipple on his or her own to breast-feed. It was first observed by a team of Swedish researchers in the 1990s who wanted to see whether newborn babies, when left alone on their mothers' abdomens, would find the breast and feed on their own. They observed that babies naturally know to crawl up the mother's abdomen to the breast, which, after a brief investigation, they latch on to and begin to suck. The baby innately knows how to find the breast. The process usually took about fifty minutes.

Later research showed that letting your baby figure out how to breast-feed on his or her own can prevent feeding problems later. Babies who self-attached had few problems latching on to the mother later, and the mothers of these babies rarely had sore nipples or breast-feeding complications. Self-attachment is now common in Norway, Sweden, and parts of Canada. Self-attachment is most successful if mother and baby are relaxed and warm, and it should be learned right after birth, if possible. If circumstances cause you to miss the chance for self-attachment at birth, you can keep trying within a few days of the birth.

The Umbilical Cord

It's common for hospitals to clamp the umbilical cord almost immediately after your baby is born. This was not a common practice until the last hundred years, and even now it's only typical in "developed" countries. Early clamping can result in shock and has been associated with brain damage and autism. In addition, it's been associated with complications fatal to infants, like hyperviscosity syndrome (blood that's too thick), infant respiratory distress, anemia, hypovolemia (not enough blood plasma), and hypoxia (oxygen deficiency).

Early clamping is dangerous, because the umbilical cord is the baby's only lifeline until he or she starts breathing. If the cord is cut before it stops pulsing, the baby's supply of oxygenated blood will be cut off. It's much safer to wait until the cord stops pulsing and the baby's lung function has been established, which will happen within about fifteen minutes after birth.

Ideally, you should wait nearly an hour, until the placenta transfusion is complete. The placenta and the umbilical cord have been part of your baby up to this point, and the blood in the placenta and the umbilical cord is your baby's blood. Think of the placenta as one of your baby's organs. It doesn't make sense to amputate a live organ! We opted to let the placenta die naturally an hour or so after birth, then severed the cord.

If the cord is not clamped too soon, the placenta gives the remaining blood it contains to the baby. Another one-third of a cup per pound is transferred within just the first three minutes after birth. This means that blood loss resulting from early clamping isn't just an effect of birth, it's your baby losing blood. In *Care in Normal Birth: A Practical Guide*, the World Health Organization acknowledges that "late clamping (or not clamping at all) is the physiological way of treating the cord, and early clamping is an intervention that needs justification."

Delaying the clamping of the umbilical cord may even boost intelligence—even a two-minute delay can boost a baby's iron level and prevent anemia for months. Infants deficient in iron display a lower cognitive ability than their iron-sufficient peers through age nineteen. We didn't clamp the umbilical cord early for either of our children. You can discuss the issue with your doctor ahead of time to make sure it doesn't happen.

If there are so many good reasons to delay clamping, why don't doctors do it? The blood passing between the baby and the placenta through the umbilical cord carries oxygen to the newborn, preventing oxygen deficiency until the baby starts breathing. Many doctors believe that inducing a shortage of oxygen will cause the baby to start breathing. This is not necessarily so.

Another common belief is that delayed clamping causes jaundice. Many midwives who practice delayed clamping haven't observed this at all. They've observed the opposite: a lower rate of jaundice when clamping is delayed. Clamping the cord is convenient for hospital procedures and speeds up the process. It's also easier for a doctor to work on a baby who's having problems if the baby isn't attached to the mother. In these situations, however, cutting the baby's life supply is probably the very worst thing the doctor could do.

Water Birth

In a water birth, the mother sits in a tub full of warm water during labor. This can reduce the pain and make the mother more comfortable. Water birth seems to help the baby into the best position for birth. Mothers like the safety of having their own place in the tub, and the warmth of the water increases the blood flow to the uterus, which increases the blood flow to the placenta and provides more oxygen for the baby.

Some women stay in the tub for the entire birthing process. If the baby is born in the tub, he or she will, of course, be brought directly to the surface before the first breath. Since your baby is still breathing through the umbilical cord, being under water for a second or two after birth isn't dangerous at all. For babies, the transition from the womb to the air is actually far more comfortable when they get to spend a few seconds in warm water.

Caesarean Section

Unless there's an emergency, we don't recommend birth by caesarean section because it is one of the most traumatic birth processes possible, for both mother and baby. A 2007 study compared the risks and benefits of caesarean birth to vaginal birth. It found that nonemergency caesarean birth results in greater risk for mother and baby regardless of a mother's medical or pregnancy history. Women having C-sections had twice the rates of illness, pregnancy-related death, hysterectomy, blood transfusion, and admission to intensive care as women having vaginal deliveries. C-sections also resulted in five times the frequency of postnatal antibiotic treatment for mothers, which is likely to result in breast milk that is less healthy and perhaps even harmful for the baby.

For the babies, caesarean delivery was associated with double the rate of staying in intensive care after birth, and neonatal death increased by 70 percent. Only in the case of breech-birth babies did caesarean section result in a lower overall risk level for both mother and baby. We know that C-sections are sometimes necessary. What we don't agree with is the widespread use of preplanned C-sections when they're not necessary. As usual, nature's way is healthier and safer most of the time. Consult your doctor and plan a vaginal delivery if you can.

Home Birth: At Least as Safe as Hospital Birth

The latest research has found home birth to be extremely safe—often safer than hospital birth. We were a little surprised to see this, and we wanted to be sure, so we looked for research that found hospital birth to be safer than home birth. But the research we found wasn't statistically sound. In one study performed in Washington, the researchers' count of home births included unplanned home births, unassisted home births, and home births in which the attendants were poorly qualified. An Australian study included high-risk home births that were far from hospitals. This study is touted by those in favor of hospital birth even though the study itself did not conclude that hospital safety statistics were higher because the births were in the hospital.

Any study tracking the safety of home versus hospital birth should consider situational circumstances that apply to most home births: they are planned and attended by a professional midwife in an area where a medical team is available within seventy-five minutes. Research has shown that mother and baby have a safety margin of about seventy-five minutes for a surgical team to arrive if there's a true emergency. In 1999 a comprehensive review was done of all studies comparing home birth to hospital birth. The authors concluded, "No evidence exists to support the claim that a hospital is the safest place for women to have normal births."

Since then, further research has only supported this finding. A 2005 study published in the *British Medical Journal* found home births and hospital births to have similar safety rates; in fact, the home births had fewer interventions and complications. A 2009 study conducted in Canada observed the outcomes of thousands of planned, midwife-assisted home births and thousands of midwife- and physician-assisted hospital births. It found that the rate of perinatal death was actually higher for hospital births than for home births. Home-born babies were less likely to need resuscitation at birth or need oxygen therapy beyond twenty-four hours of age. While home birth presented no increased risk for the babies, the mothers actually benefited greatly from it. The women who had planned home births were far less likely to have obstetric interventions or adverse maternal outcomes like third- or fourth-degree perineal tears.

The Issue of Hospital Birth

When we thought about birth from the perspective of epigenetics, it became clear why hospital birth is riskier than home birth these days. Hospital births are rife with unnecessary interventions that create stress for both mother and baby, often traumatic stress. In short, hospital births are often far from gentle.

Unnecessary C-sections, epidurals, Pitocin (a drug used to induce contractions), and intravenous drugs are used in hospital births every day. Many of these procedures are toxic or otherwise harmful for a baby, especially during birth, which even under ideal conditions is a situation of extreme stress and even clinical shock for a baby. Epidurals can lower the mother's blood pressure so much that the baby is getting far less oxygen through the placenta, which can cause fetal distress and require an emergency C-section.

Pitocin can cause uterine contractions so strong they induce fetal distress, which can derail the baby's growth mode during his or her emergence into the world, one of the most critical developmental stages. The intravenous narcotic drugs given to mothers to relieve their pain affect the baby so much that he or she may not even begin breathing after birth. For this condition, there's yet another drug that hospitals use to get the baby to start breathing.

At home, women are free to give birth in positions that minimize stress on the baby: squatting, on hands and knees, or in a tub of warm water. Compare this with the stressful and painful position commonly used in hospitals, in which the woman lies on her back in the hospital bed (making birth occur against the force of gravity rather than with it). Birthing at home also gives the family members the chance to exercise their own desires or customs, such as the father catching the baby or the siblings being involved.

Beyond having to endure interference and drugs, babies born in hospitals get infections four times as often as home-born babies, and those infections are more likely to be resistant to antibiotic treatment. This is serious, considering that more people (ninety thousand a year) die from hospital-acquired infections than from all accidental deaths combined (seventy thousand a year), including automobile crashes, fires, burns, falls, drownings, and poisonings. Another ninety-eight thousand people die every year from medical errors.

Mothers giving birth in hospitals are cared for by so many different people that the potential for miscommunication among them is great. One hospital even released a report detailing how a baby died as a result of miscommunication among hospital personnel. Many people are convinced that a hospital must be the safest place to give birth to a baby because of all of the equipment that's available. Yet if you are having a normal delivery, you do not need that equipment. And unless the right people are there to use the equipment, it's not helpful.

Most women go into labor at night. This is the time of day when there are fewer registered nurses and trained physicians available to use this equipment and more medical technicians are on duty, and they often know *how* to use the equipment but not necessarily *when*. A 2005 study found that a higher rate of neonatal death for babies born at night, and staff availability is a reasonable cause.

Many hospitals separate the mother and the baby almost immediately after birth. From the perspective of epigenetics, this is a life-changing disruption of the natural growth processes in the baby. This separation also deprives mothers of the nipple stimulation from immediate nursing that they need to release oxytocin naturally. Making things worse, as we noted earlier, most hospitals clamp the umbilical cord within seconds of birth, cutting off the baby's life supply.

Oxytocin is a hormone that plays a large role in female reproduction and birth. Immediately after birth, oxytocin is responsible for contracting the uterus and preventing postpartum hemorrhage. Although hospitals now use synthetic oxytocin to control this, we're certain that separating the mother from the baby is ultimately detrimental to both, especially if the oxytocin is not bioidentical. Babies also release oxytocin from early contact with their mothers, raising their body temperatures to deal with the new, cooler environment of the outside world.

A 1998 study pointed out that contact with the mother is a more effective way to warm a baby than an incubator is. Many hospitals bathe the newborns so soon that the babies' body temperatures become dangerously low. Hospitals engaging in this practice do so against the World Health Organization's recommendation that a baby not be bathed for six hours after birth.

Considering all of this, it seems that hospitals have little regard for the fact that they're dealing with a critical time in a new baby's life and that their practices are often at the mother's expense rather than for her benefit. Countries with the very safest maternity care don't use risky medical procedures unless absolutely necessary. The five European countries with the lowest infant mortality rates—Iceland, Sweden, Finland, Norway, Luxembourg—use midwives for more than 70 percent of births. In the Netherlands, more than half of the babies are born at home assisted by a professional midwife. Their infant mortality rate is far lower than the rate in the United States, where hospital birth is predominant.

Lana, who comes from Sweden, was shocked to see the heavy interference in the birth process in the United States. Here birth is viewed as
a medical emergency right from the outset. In Sweden, birth is viewed as
a natural bodily process that works best with no interference except in
serious emergencies. Scheduled C-sections, for nonmedical reasons, are
fairly common in the United States but nonexistent in Sweden. In
Scandinavia, and most of Europe, a C-section is properly viewed for
what it is: major abdominal surgery. So it is performed only when indicated on serious medical grounds. Even women who live very far away
from a hospital or a birthing center will not have a scheduled C-section.
They are just admitted well ahead of time, so they can deliver naturally.

Planning Birth at Home or in the Hospital

Now that you're aware of what makes for a gentle birth and what makes
conventional hospital birth so harsh for mother and baby, you can take
steps to plan for a gentle birth, whether you choose home or the hospital
for your location.

We chose to plan birth at home because we wanted to have full
control over the birth environment so we could take each of the steps
discussed above without any interference or mistakes in communication among hospital staff. We worked with our midwife, Ronnie, from
the moment of conception and carefully arranged for backup care from
a local hospital if necessary, especially since Lana was over thirty-five,
the age at which risks start to go up significantly. After going through
two home births, we're happy we chose that. Lana found it very com-
forting to be surrounded by familiar faces, and she really appreciated
having the greatest comfort and privacy possible. Ultimately though,
you will have the best birth in the place where you feel most comfortable and safe. If this is in the hospital, here's a checklist of things to
create gentle birth:

- If you're working with a midwife, you can request that your midwife be the primary birth assistant in the hospital and that your
  doctor be available as medical backup.
- Insist that no drugs be used unless *you* ask for them, or there is a
  medical emergency.

- Ask the hospital staff to let you give birth in the position you're most comfortable with. You might even request a water birth.

- Ask the staff not to separate you from your baby after birth or bathe your baby too early.

- Ask the staff not to clamp the umbilical cord until you give permission.

- As soon as it's confirmed that you and your baby are okay, ensure that privacy will be granted.

- Have a C-section only if it's an absolute emergency. Many doctors in the United States will do an unplanned and unnecessary C-section in the heat of the moment, so this is something you'll want to plan well in advance and make sure your doctor understands.

- If the hospital won't grant all of your requests, you can look for another hospital, a birthing center, or consider home birth.

A European Perspective on Birth

As a Swedish doctor, Lana is amazed at the difference in the ways that birth is viewed and dealt with in the United States and in Sweden (and Europe in general). In the United States, a profound mistrust of the natural birth process is prevalent. The planned C-sections, frivolous interventions, and heavy regimen of vaccinations within a few days of birth are unnatural and uncommon in other parts of the world. Also, maternity leave from employment is extremely short in the United States.

In Sweden, most births are assisted by midwives in hospitals or birthing centers attached to hospitals. An ob-gyn will be present only if there is a serious complication or a medical emergency. There are few C-sections and other interventions, and there certainly aren't any planned convenience C-sections. Maternity leave from employment in Sweden starts an entire month before the due date, and a partial salary can extend up to eighteen months after birth. In Germany and the Netherlands, home births are very common.

The postpartum bonding of mother and baby is considered very important in Sweden; the mother and the baby are not separated right after birth unless there is a life-threatening emergency. Nurses in maternity wards are encouraged not to handle the baby, and the father is encouraged to catch the baby and hand him or her to the mother, so frequently a baby has been touched only by his or her parents within the first few hours of birth. The baby is not washed or weighed until he or she is fully acclimated to life outside the womb. Swedes would be absolutely shocked to hear that babies in the United States are given silver nitrate eyedrops and shots of vitamin K right after birth. The heel prick test where blood is taken from the baby's heel with a sharp lancet is done when a baby is five days old, not right after birth. Vaccines are nowhere in sight at the maternity ward. The Swedish vaccination program, like many other European programs, starts at three months of age. Only then is a baby considered old enough to have developed the beginnings of an immune system and therefore able to benefit from the vaccines.

Planning a Vaginal Birth after a Caesarian

Many women who have had a C-section wish to have a vaginal birth later. This is called *vaginal birth after caesarian*, or VBAC. Generally, VBACs are considered safe unless a woman has had two C-sections before and has never given birth vaginally or if there is scarring above the lower, thinner part of the uterus. Only your doctor can tell you whether VBAC will be safe for you, given your individual condition. If after consulting with your doctor you decide to plan a VBAC, it's a smart move to take extra steps to strengthen your uterine and vaginal tissues. Although there's no study proving that poor nutrition results in a greater incidence of uterine rupture, a weaker uterus would of course be more likely to rupture. And just as a malnourished body is weaker in general, so is a malnourished uterus.

The methods that strengthen the uterus involve the same foods and supplements we use for so many other reasons. Taken in the last trimester, hydrolyzed collagen and glycine give the body the raw protein materials it needs to strengthen the tissues. Vitamin C (five thousand milligrams a day), N-acetyl cysteine, and a high-quality liposomal glutathione will keep the tissues detoxified, which is paramount when

strengthening tissue. Fresh vegetables provide a range of enzymes, vitamins, and minerals that the body needs to build and detox the tissues.
Taken throughout pregnancy, these foods and supplements will go a long
way toward preventing uterine rupture.

Mycotoxins can be a grave threat for VBAC, because they disrupt
endocrine function and damage the reproductive system. Activated charcoal, bentonite and zeolite clays, and carrots can help the body to eliminate mycotoxins. If you've had a C-section before, taking these steps at
any time will strengthen the reproductive organs. Ideally, you should plan
to strengthen them before you become pregnant again.

Nursing

There's now an overwhelming amount of research proving that breast
feeding helps your baby to grow his or her very best, far outperforming
formula in a number of areas, including brain development.

A 1999 study led by James W. Anderson of the University of
Kentucky drew on twenty previous studies on cognitive development
scores since 1929, only ten of which were done in the United States.
Dr. Anderson's study concluded that "breast-feeding was associated
with significantly higher scores for cognitive development than was
formula feeding." The breast-fed children had an average IQ that was
2.7 to 5 points higher than the average IQ of the formula-fed children.
The children who were born with a lower birth weight saw a greater
intelligence increase from breast-feeding than children who were born
at a normal birth weight. In addition, the children who were breast-fed
for longer than twenty-eight weeks outperformed children who were
breast-fed for eight to eleven weeks and strongly outperformed formula-
fed children.

In the twenty studies combined, the intelligence tests were performed
on children who ranged from six months to sixteen years of age, so the
effects were observed over a wide range of ages and maturity levels;
regardless of age, breast-fed children outperformed their formula-fed
counterparts. This was true whether the formulas contained added
omega-3 or not.

Breast milk has other advantages over manufactured formulas. First, formula couldn't possibly replace the mother's colostrum, which is very high in antibodies to jump-start her baby's immune system. No formula manufacturer could anticipate the exact set of antibodies a baby will need most, but the mother's body knows exactly how to protect the baby.

Second, breast milk is easier to digest, and we're sure that breast milk contains many things that we cannot reproduce and add to baby formulas. During a critical time of development, a formula-fed baby is deprived of much of the raw materials he or she needs to develop properly. From an epigenetics perspective, the act of breast-feeding can itself activate infant growth genes. No formula can replicate this.

Eating Right to Make Healthy Milk

The essential fatty acid content of mother's milk is heavily dependent on the mother's own diet. This means that until you're done nursing (preferably not till after twelve to eighteen months), you should continue to eat a diet high in healthy fats and low in unhealthy ones. Eating right for nursing is just like eating right for pregnancy. If you're following the diet we describe in this book, your milk will be rich in all of the nutrients your baby needs. As always, the healthy fats are important, because breast milk is 50 percent fat by calorie, with half of that being saturated fat. About 18 percent of the saturated fats are medium-chain triglycerides (MCTs), like what is found in coconut oil. To maintain the right healthy fat levels in your milk, eat these foods on a daily basis:

- Two raw egg yolks
- One serving of krill oil capsules
- Two tablespoons of cold-pressed walnut, almond, or nut oil for omega-3
- Three to four tablespoons of coconut cream, meat, or oil, or a high-quality MCT oil
- Plenty of full-fat butter produced exclusively from 100 percent grass-fed cows (any other butter will be far too high in omega-6)
- Five tablespoons of cold-pressed olive oil (for no more than seven grams of omega-6)

Considering all of the healthy fat you'll be eating during pregnancy, your body will long be accustomed to this kind of fat intake. To learn more about other sources of healthy fats like avocados, see chapter 5.

Formula has many shortcomings. One of its greatest faults is its lack of healthy fats. We know that breast-milk is 50 percent fat and that the nonwater makeup of the brain is more than 60 percent fat. We also know that if a baby doesn't consume enough fat, his or her brain is not likely to be constructed to its fullest potential. Breast milk is high in DHA and ALA, two fatty acids that compose a large amount of the brain's fat. Even though some of the better brands of formula now contain DHA and ALA, they still lack many of the essential fatty acids contained in a mother's milk. In addition, the DHA and ALA in these formulas come from microalgae and are oxidized (toxic).

What If Breastfeeding Isn't an Option?

Although infant health and cognitive development is best supported by breast-feeding, there are some situations in which breast milk may be unavailable. For these times, and for these times only, we suggest a recipe to fortify a standard high-end formula with extra nutrients. It's the best alternative we've found. All of this comes with the caveat, however, that if you are able to breast-feed your baby, you are doing him or her a great disservice if you choose not to. Also, try to get breast milk from a lactating friend or family member before you use formula. Formula should be the very last resort.

When you must use formula, here is how you can fortify a high-quality one with the fatty acids it lacks. This recipe is derived from a Weston A. Price Foundation recipe.

> 1 cup milk-based powdered formula, preferably Nutramigen or Alimentum—infants tolerate them better than other formulas. Make sure it is organic and free of soy.
>
> 29 ounces filtered water (3 5/8 cups)
>
> 1 large raw organic egg yolk
>
> 1 capsule krill oil or ½ teaspoon cod liver oil
>
> organic cream, nonpasteurized and nonhomogenized (raw)

1 teaspoon Omega Nutrition brand pure sesame, walnut, safflower, and sunflower oils (rotate these four)

1 teaspoon high-quality mycotoxin-free coconut oil

Place all ingredients (including the contents of the krill oil capsule, not the capsule itself) in a blender or a food processor and blend thoroughly. Place six to eight ounces in a clean glass bottle and store the rest in the refrigerator. To feed the baby, attach a clean nipple to the bottle and set in a pan of simmering water until the formula is warm but not hot. Heating the formula too much will denature the casein in the organic cream, which would be unhealthy.

What Not to Feed Your Baby

If you're not breast-feeding your baby and you're using the recipe above, it's important to use a high-quality commercial formula like Nutramigen or Alimentum as the base. These two brands of formula cause fewer allergic reactions in infants than other formulas. It's a bad idea to make your own base formula or create your own base formula recipe. Without the exact right blend, your baby could be getting too much of one substance or not enough of another. Although high-quality formulas are no replacement for real breast milk, manufacturers have done lots of research to design formulas that keep your baby alive and growing, so it's wise to start with a quality commercial formula.

You may have heard that soy milk, almond milk, and carrot juice are good substitutes for breast milk. This isn't true. Even if they're organic, they're not sufficient replacements for commercial formula, let alone breast milk.

Soy-based formulas are damaging and dangerous for infants. Never feed your baby soy. Soy is so high in manganese, aluminum, and phytoestrogens that soy formula isn't safe for infants. A recent study has linked ADHD with high levels of manganese. Breast milk contains only four to six micrograms per liter of manganese, whereas milk-based formulas contain thirty to fifty. Soy formulas contain an astounding two to three hundred! Two popular soy-based formulas are Isomil by Ross Products and ProSobee by Mead Johnson. Some manganese is essential for life and is used in cell energy production, but in high quantities, manganese is a known neurotoxin.

Vaccines

Vaccination has become a hot topic in recent years as provaccine and antivaccine groups have promoted their positions in the media and through research. We did our own research, and we believe the best approach is to avoid vaccines at least for the first several years of a child's life. Neurotoxic heavy metals are used as preservatives and adjuvants in the vaccines, and now that we have epigenetics to guide us, we know all too well how these toxins can disrupt a child's growth, especially at critical stages like right after birth. The most prevalent toxins in vaccines are heavy metals, like the preservative thimerosal and the aluminum salts that are used as an adjuvant.

Even conventional medicine rarely recommends vaccines to pregnant women. Stimulating a pregnant mother's immune system during midterm or late-term pregnancy is linked to much higher rates of autism and schizophrenia. The Gardasil vaccine for cervical cancer is a perfect example of why avoiding vaccines during pregnancy is a good idea regardless of what you're told.

When Gardasil was released, both the Centers for Disease Control and Merck, the maker of the vaccine, recommended that pregnant women get the vaccine in the first trimester. Shortly thereafter, this recommendation was swiftly withdrawn, because women who got the vaccine started miscarrying or giving birth to babies with major malformations. Some may fret and wonder how this happened, but unfortunately it makes perfect sense. Gardasil contains amorphous aluminum hydroxyphosphate.

Some vaccines are very poorly tested before being touted to the public as safe and effective. In 2009, the H1N1 swine flu vaccine was declared safe after people who received the vaccine in testing were observed for a mere seven days. But neurotoxic effects like seizures, behavioral problems, and autism could become manifest years later.

18

Bringing It All Together

It would be nearly impossible to condense *The Better Baby Book* into a single chapter without losing important information, yet this chapter exists for prospective parents who are simply so eager to get started that they have not yet read the entire book. It is also here as a reminder of the most important things you can do before and during pregnancy to increase the odds of having a healthier, smarter baby.

This summary only includes what to do; the reasons these techniques work are spread throughout the book. We sincerely hope you will take the time to read the entire book and to use it to improve your health, your children's health, and even your grandchildren's health.

Getting the Right Stuff into Your Body

Too often people make the mistake of choosing an unhealthy food because it contains some healthy nutrient or another. Other times, they believe health myths, like the idea that cutting calories will lead to health.

Eat the Right Foods and Skip the Toxins

Simply following the Better Baby diet will do wonders for helping your body to restore and maintain healthy hormone levels, and it will provide the right building blocks for making the healthiest baby you can. The diet also automatically helps you to choose foods that have fewer hidden toxins and antinutrients in them. Toxins hidden in food can have a much larger effect on fertility and pregnancy outcome than most people ever imagine. Always eat organic food when you can. Never eat factory-farmed (nonorganic) animals, because they are usually fattened with synthetic estrogen or antibiotics that remain in the meat.

Take a Good Multivitamin

Good nutritional supplementation requires more than a single pill per day to fit in all the nutrients your body needs. We have recommended brands on our website, at www.betterbabybook.com/supplements. Look for up to 50 milligrams of vitamin B6 and extra iron. Look for at least 500 milligrams of vitamin C. We recommend taking folinic acid, a more available and nontoxic form of folic acid, at 4,000 micrograms or more per day. Avoid more than 8,000 international units of preformed vitamin A (retinol), because it blocks vitamin D3. At least 400 milligrams of magnesium daily is also very important.

Take Vitamin C

Lana took at most 8 grams per day of vitamin C divided into at least two doses per day before and throughout her pregnancies, largely because of a 1971 *Journal of Applied Nutrition* report by Frederick R. Klenner, M.D. Dr. Klenner reports, "Observations made on over 300 consecutive obstetrical cases using supplemental ascorbic acid, by mouth, convinced me that failure to use this agent in sufficient amounts in pregnancy borders on malpractice." His studies of three hundred pregnancy outcomes used a program of 4 grams of vitamin C per day in the first trimester, 6 grams per day in the second, and 10 grams per day in the third trimester, with some women receiving up to 15 grams per day of vitamin C. The results were impressive. There was a large reduction in problems with leg cramps, blood iron levels, stretch marks, delivery, post-birth healing, and baby health. In fact, this vitamin C program led to the first successful birth of quadruplets in the Southeast United States.

There are rumors on the Internet about vitamin C causing miscarriage. We've done extensive searching, and there appears to be no conclusive evidence that vitamin C causes abortions or prevents pregnancy. However, there is a reasonable theory that suddenly starting or stopping large doses of vitamin C during pregnancy could potentially be harmful to a pregnancy. For this reason, Lana made sure to take vitamin C on a daily basis while pregnant.

Take Vitamin D3

Take 1,000 international units of vitamin D3 for every twenty-five pounds of body weight. Better yet, get an affordable blood test to see how much you need to be taking. Getting your vitamin D level right is one of the most affordable, effective things you can do for your baby.

Take Krill Oil and DHA Fish Oil

Take up to 10 grams (¾ tablespoon) of DHA-rich, mercury-free fish oil per day. Do not exceed this dose. Also take 500 milligrams of krill oil. Back off on both of these if you experience any unusual bleeding, and stop completely a week before your due date.

Take Collagen Protein

Collagen is one of the most important types of protein in the body; it provides a scaffolding for the bones and organs in growing bodies. Modern diets are deficient in collagen. We recommend at least ten grams per day.

Test Your Thyroid

It is shockingly common for women to have slightly underactive thyroid glands even in the face of "normal" results from a family physician. Pregnancy can also cause thyroid problems. If your thyroid level is low, your baby will be less healthy and potentially even less intelligent. Warning signs include dry skin and thin hair, constipation, and always feeling cold. Even if you don't have those symptoms, having your thyroid checked and treated if necessary can do wonders for fertility and for pregnancy health. Look for a thyroid-stimulating hormone level of three or less before pregnancy, and even lower during pregnancy. Make sure you have your T3 and T4 levels checked at the same time. They should be mid to high normal. If you're already on thyroid medication, your doctor should raise the dosage during pregnancy.

Keep the Bad Stuff Out

When you're pregnant, it's much more important to avoid toxins than it normally is. A fetus is very susceptible to a variety of toxins, and many of these are active at very small doses. Follow our advice in the book to learn how to avoid most of them.

Follow the Better Baby Diet

Our diet is designed to keep food toxins at bay while providing maximum nutrition for a growing baby and mother. Be scrupulous about avoiding gluten (wheat) and cooked dairy products, except butter. Wheat and milk are linked to a whole host of epigenetic (multigenerational) problems.

Stop Drinking Alcohol and Avoid Coffee and Tea

Even one drink of alcohol a day can increase ovulatory infertility by 30 percent, and fetal alcohol syndrome is a well-known problem. Most women know to stop drinking coffee when they're pregnant, but many switch to green tea instead. Green tea dramatically increases your need for folic acid, so limit your intake to one cup per day and increase your folinic acid supplements if you drink it.

Detox Your Home and Skip the Nursery

Household chemicals are a major source of pollution in the average home. Switch to organic cleaners and personal care products. Avoid air fresheners and pesticides. If you've had any chronic health problems, test the air in your home for the presence of mold spores. A moldy home has the potential to cause autism, and homes with mold are surprisingly more common than you'd think. We estimate that many houses may have problems that could affect a pregnancy.

If you must prepare a nursery, at least use nontoxic paints. When the mommy hormones kick in, there is a powerful urge to nest. For us humans, that means preparing a nursery, often with toxic paint, furniture, and carpet. You don't want to deal with those added toxins while you're pregnant. Hang a mobile and some pretty colorful silks, and your baby will be perfectly happy for the first year.

Manage Stress

A mother's stress hormones have a lifelong impact on her baby's health. It is critical to manage the stress pregnant women feel, but it's easier to say that than it is to figure out how to actually manage stress. Here's how we do it.

Meditation with Heart Rate Variability

Lots of mothers manage stress using meditation. If this works for you, keep doing it. We find that many people believe they are meditating properly but that they are not getting the benefits in the form of a lowered stress level. There is a small device called the emWave from the Institute of Heart Math in California that makes it very easy to calm stress in the body. It pairs deep-breathing exercises with a light that turns green when you are in the best state for managing your stress. This state, called coherence, is also pleasant for babies to experience in the womb. Getting even ten minutes of this type of biofeedback every day before and during pregnancy can work miracles on stress. (Dave is a certified Heart Math coach!)

Sleep

Sleep is incredibly important for managing stress hormones. Before and during your pregnancy, make every effort to get a full night's sleep, and be sure your bedroom is completely dark.

Giving Birth at Home

It is stressful for a mother and her baby to sit in the hospital with flashing lights and beeping equipment and nurses and doctors rushing around. There is evidence that a calm, safe birthing environment leads to more comfortable mothers and less stressed babies. For normal pregnancies, a competent midwife can provide the same level of safety you would find in a hospital. Birth should be a beautiful, emotional experience, not a medical emergency or a surgical procedure. A calm birth in a comfortable familiar environment can do wonders for mother and baby alike.

Travel

Minimize long trips in the car and especially airplane flights. This gets more important later in the pregnancy, but long days of travel (especially when a change in time zones is involved) can cause a lot of stress on the body and the mind. Pregnancy is not the time for that kind of stress.

Exercise

Before you conceive, focus on building strength and endurance by doing high-intensity weight-bearing exercise for at most twenty minutes twice a week, or do interval training if you're already a runner. Avoid daily long cardio sessions lasting more than forty-five minutes, because these raise your stress-hormone levels and do not deliver much benefit compared to the T-Tapp exercises we recommend. After you're pregnant, lower the intensity and weight. Your baby, not you, should be putting on muscle!

An exercise program that is excellent during early pregnancy is Teresa Tapp's fifteen-minute workout. This is a form of aerobic exercise that leads to visible reductions in back fat and "love handles" in just days. It's the most powerful detoxing workout we could find, because it focuses on circulating the lymph. We recommend doing T-Tapp at least four times per week before you conceive and during the first trimester, but not during the second or third. We provide links to appropriate T-Tapp exercises at www.betterbabybook.com/exercise.

Yoga is good exercise and can be done throughout pregnancy, although pregnancy yoga is more gentle than normal yoga. Yoga helps you to relax and feel good. It's good for the mind and the body, and many mothers have found that it helps enormously. We did, too.

For Men

It turns out that the health of the father in the months before conception has a large effect on the baby's health for life. Men should take more vitamin C than women: more than 1,000 milligrams per day in divided doses. The amino acids L-arginine (5 grams, taken at night) and acetyl L-carnitine (1 or 2 grams, taken in the morning) can build healthier sperm, and so can 200 milligrams of the best form of selenium, seleno-methionine, taken with 50 milligrams of zinc.

Your Beautiful Better Baby

There is something else that's more important than everything on this list, and that is love. When a woman or an unborn baby feels a lack of love and support, it creates psychological and epigenetic effects that last for generations. Fix your relationships before you get pregnant. If you're already pregnant and in a bad relationship, do what will lower your stress the most while you're pregnant.

Keep in mind that you don't have to do even one thing in this book in order to have a beautiful, healthy, very intelligent baby. No one is perfect, and seeking perfection with the Better Baby Plan will only make you feel stressed. When you use this book as a guide to make healthier decisions every day, you'll feel better, your pregnancy will most likely get easier, and your baby will have a head start on a healthy life. Aside from a parent's love, no greater gift can be given to a child than a strong body and a healthy brain.

Index